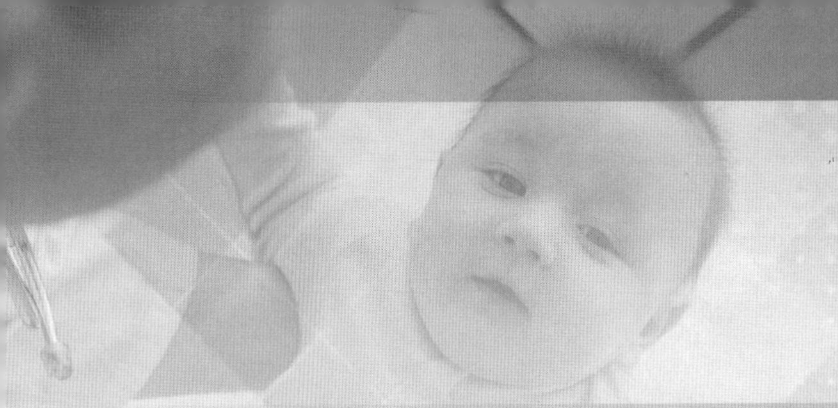

Practical Record Book of

Child Health Nursing

For GNM Nursing Students

(As per the New Syllabus of INC for GNM)

Nursing Knowledge Tree
An Initiative by CBS Nursing Division

Practical Record Book of

Child Health Nursing

For GNM Nursing Students

(As per the New Syllabus of INC for GNM)

Second Edition

Neeti Sharma MSc (Pediatric Nursing)
Nursing Officer
Dr Yashwant Singh Parmar Government Medical College
Nahan, Himachal Pradesh, India

CBSPD
Dedicated to Education

CBS Publishers & Distributors Pvt Ltd

• New Delhi • Bengaluru • Chennai • Kochi • Kolkata • Lucknow • Mumbai
• Hyderabad • Jharkhand • Nagpur • Patna • Pune • Uttarakhand

Practical Record Book of

Child Health Nursing

For GNM Nursing Students

(As per the New Syllabus of INC for GNM)

ISBN: 978-93-94525-64-1

Reprint: 2026

Second Edition: 2024

First Edition: 2018

Published by **Satish Kumar Jain** and produced by **Varun Jain** for

CBS Publishers & Distributors Pvt Ltd
4819/XI Prahlad Street, 24 Ansari Road, Daryaganj, New Delhi 110 002, India.
Ph: +91-11-23289259, 23266861, 23266867 Website: www.cbspd.com
Fax: 011-23243014
e-mail: delhi@cbspd.com; cbspubs@airtelmail.in.

Corporate Office: 204 FIE, Industrial Area, Patparganj, Delhi 110 092
Ph: +91-11-4934 4934 Fax: 4934 4935
e-mail: feedback@cbspd.com; bhupesharora@cbspd.com

Branches

- **Bengaluru:** Seema House 2975, 17th Cross, K.R. Road, Banashankari 2nd Stage, Bengaluru-560 070, Karnataka
  Ph: +91-80-26771678/79 Fax: +91-80-26771680 e-mail: bangalore@cbspd.com
- **Chennai:** 7, Subbaraya Street, Shenoy Nagar, Chennai-600 030, Tamil Nadu
  Ph: +91-44-26680620, 26681266 Fax: +91-44-42032115 e-mail: chennai@cbspd.com
- **Kochi:** 68/1534, 35, 36-Power House Road, Opp. KSEB, Cochin-682018, Kochi, Kerala
  Ph: +91-484-4059061-65 Fax: +91-484-4059065 e-mail: kochi@cbspd.com
- **Kolkata:** Hind Ceramics Compound, 1st Floor, 147, Nilganj Road, Belghoria, Kolkata-700056, West Bengal
  Ph: +033-2563-3055/56 e-mail: kolkata@cbspd.com
- **Lucknow:** Basement, Khushnuma Complex, 7-Meerabai Marg (Behind Jawahar Bhawan), Lucknow-226001, Uttar Pradesh
  Ph: +0522-4000032 e-mail: tiwari.lucknow@cbspd.com
- **Mumbai:** PWD Shed, Gala No. 25/26, Ramchandra Bhatt Marg, Next to J.J. Hospital Gate No. 2, Opp. Union Bank of India, Noor Baug, Mumbai-400009, Maharashtra
  Ph: +91-22-66661880/89 Fax: +91-22-24902342 e-mail: mumbai@cbspd.com

Representatives

- **Hyderabad** +91-9885175004
- **Jharkhand** +91-9811541605
- **Nagpur** +91-9421945513
- **Patna** +91-9334159340
- **Pune** +91-9623451994
- **Uttarakhand** +91-9716462459

Printed at : Goyal Offset Works Pvt. Ltd. Haryana

Preface

I am overwhelmed to present the second edition of the Practical Record Book of *Child Health Nursing for GNM Nursing Students*. Building on the success of the previous edition, this updated version aims to provide an even more comprehensive and user-friendly resource for GNM Nursing Students in Pediatric Nursing.

While crafting this revised edition, I have meticulously aligned the evaluation criteria with the latest guidelines from the syllabus of Indian Nursing Council (INC). The content formats are designed to facilitate a thorough assessment of students, ensuring their proficiency in Child Health Nursing.

We have taken into consideration the invaluable feedback received from educators, students, and practitioners who utilized the previous edition. Your insights have been instrumental in refining and enhancing the content to meet the evolving needs of nursing education.

I extend my sincere gratitude to all those who have contributed to the success of the previous edition and invite continued collaboration. Your comments and suggestions are invaluable in maintaining the accuracy and quality of this record book.

Feel free to reach out to me at sharmaneeti8509@gmail.com with any feedback, corrections, or ideas for further improvement.

I hope that this revised edition continues to serve as a valuable companion for GNM Nursing Students, aiding them in their journey toward excellence in Child Health Nursing. Thank you for your ongoing support and commitment to the advancement of nursing education.

Neeti Sharma

Acknowledgments

I am grateful to my family and friends for supporting and helping in completing this project. I also express heart-felt gratitude to my in-laws and my husband (Manan) for their constant support and motivation and my daughter Shambhvi who keeps my spirit alive for work. I also thank my parents who have toiled to make me what I am today.

I would like to thank **Mr Satish Kumar Jain** (Chairman) and **Mr Varun Jain** (Managing Director), M/s CBS Publishers and Distributors Pvt Ltd for providing me the platform in bringing out the book. I have no words to describe the role, efforts, inputs and initiatives undertaken by **Mr Bhupesh Aarora** [Sr. Vice President – Publishing and Marketing (Health Sciences Division)] for helping and motivating me.

I sincerely thank the entire CBS team for bringing out the book with utmost care and attractive presentation. I would like to thank Ms Nitasha Arora (Assistant General Manager Publishing – Medical and Nursing), and Dr Anju Dhir (Sr. Product Manager and Medical Development Editor) for their publishing support. I would also extend my thanks to Ms Surbhi Gupta, Team Lead (Editorial), Mr Ashutosh Pathak (Assistant Production Manager) and all the production team members for devoting laborious hours in editing, designing and typesetting the book.

CBSPD

Dedicated to Education

Nursing Knowledge Tree

CBS Nursing Knowledge Tree

Extends its Tribute to

Florence Nightingale

For glorifying the role of women as nurses,
For holding the title of " The Lady with the Lamp,"
For working tirelessly for humanity–
Florence Nightingale will always be
remembered for her
selfless and memorable services to the
human race.

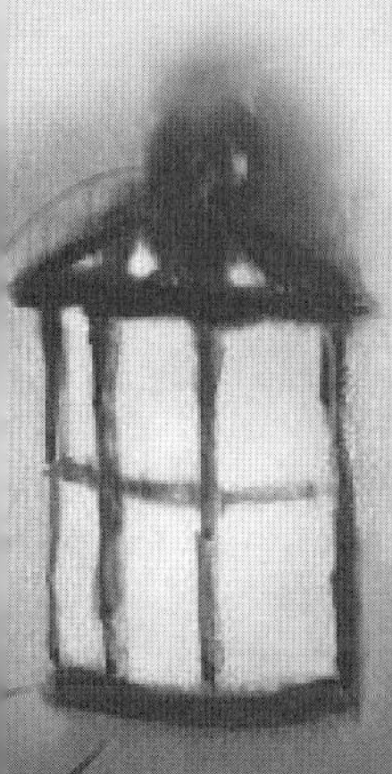

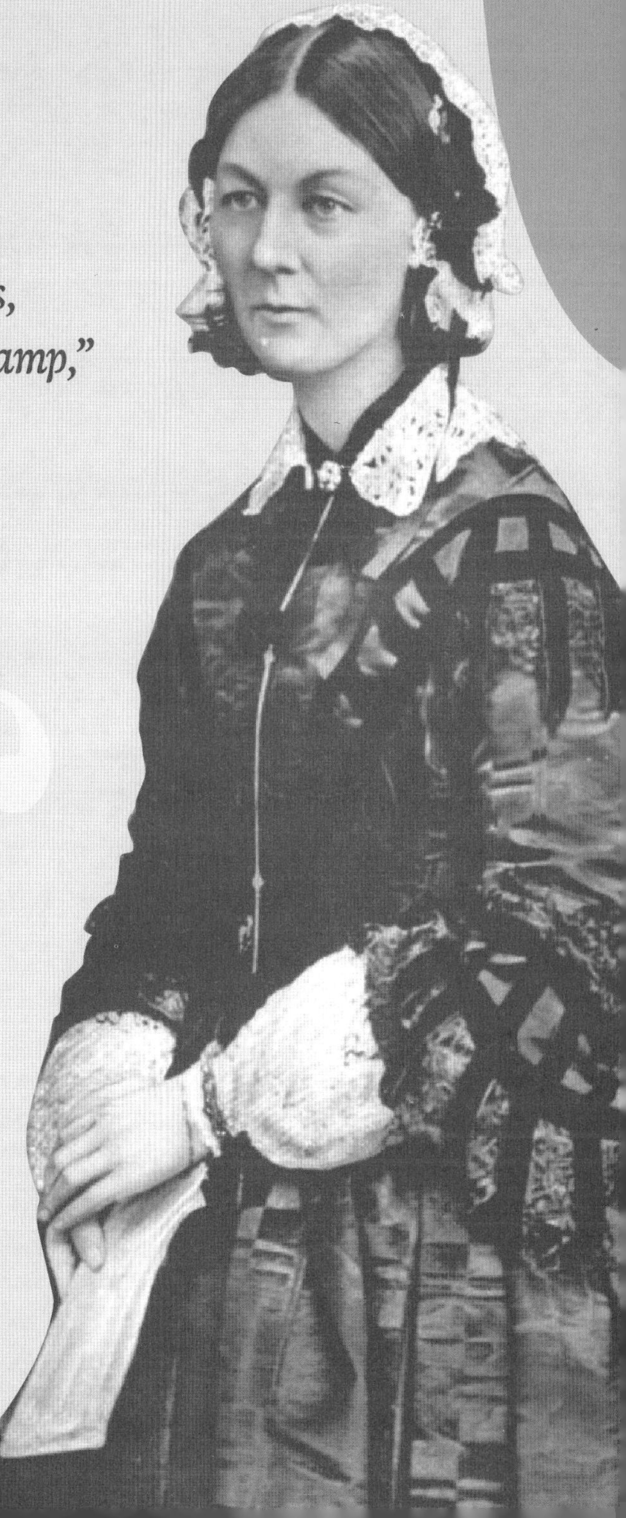

Florence Nightingale
(May 1820 – August 1910)

From the Publisher's Desk

Dear Reader,

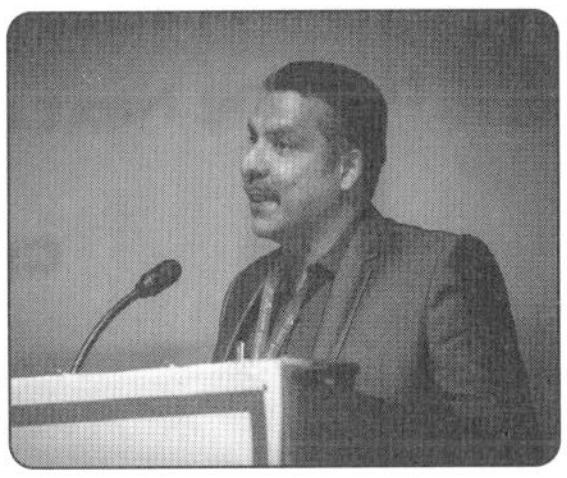

Nursing Education has a rich history, often characterized by traditional teaching techniques that have evolved over time. Primarily, teaching took place within classroom settings. Lectures, textbooks, and clinical rotations were the core teaching tools; and students majorly relied on textbooks by local or foreign publishers for quality education. However, today, technology has completely transformed the field of nursing education, making it an integral part of the curriculum. It has evolved to include a range of technological tools that enhance the learning experience and better prepare students for clinical practice.

As publishers, we've been contributing to the field of Medical Science, Nursing and Allied Sciences and earned the trust of many. By supporting **Indian authors**, coupled with **nursing webinars and conferences**, we have paved an easier path for aspiring nurses, empowering them to excel in national and state level exams. With this, we're not only enhancing the quality of patient care but also enabling future nurses to adapt to new challenges and innovations in the rapidly evolving world of healthcare. Following the ideology of **Bringing learning to people instead of people going for learning**, so far, we've been doing our part by:

- Developing quality content by qualified and well-versed authors
- Building a strong community of faculty and students
- Introducing a smart approach with Digital/Hybrid Books, and
- Offering simulation Nursing Procedures, etc.

Innovative teaching methodologies, such as modern-age Phygital Books, have sparked the interest of the Next-Gen students in pursuing advanced education. The enhancement of educational standards through **Omnipresent Knowledge Sharing Platforms** has further facilitated learning, bridging the gap between doctors and nurses.

At Nursing Next Live, a sister concern of CBS Publishers & Distributors, we have long recognized the immense potential within the nursing field. Our journey in innovating nursing education has allowed us to make substantial and meaningful contributions. With the vision of strengthening learning at every stage, we have introduced several plans that cater to the specific needs of the students, including but not limited to **Plan UG** for undergraduates, **Plan MSc** for postgraduate aspirants, **Plan FDP** for upskilling faculties, **SDL** for integrated learning and **Plan NP** for bridging the gap between theoretical & practical learning. Additionally, we have successfully completed seven series of our **Target High** Book in a very short period, setting a milestone in the education industry. We have been able to achieve all this just with the sole vision of laying the foundation of diversified knowledge for all. With the rise of a new generation of educated, tech-savvy individuals, we anticipate even more remarkable advancements in the coming years.

We take immense pride in our achievements and eagerly look forward to the future, brimming with new opportunities for innovation, growth and collaborations with experienced minds such as yourself who can contribute to our mission as Authors, Reviewers and/or Faculties. Together, let's foster a generation of nurses who are confident, competent, and prepared to succeed in a technology-driven healthcare system.

Mr Bhupesh Aarora
(Sr Vice President – Publishing & Marketing)
bhupeshaarora@cbspd.com| +91 95553 53330

Syllabus

CHILD HEALTH NURSING

PRACTICAL

Time: 320 hours (8 weeks)
Internship: 96 hours (2 weeks)

Placement: Third Year

Areas	Duration	Objectives	Skill	Assignment	Assessment Methods
Pediatric medicine ward	3 weeks	• Perform physical assessment • Assist in diagnostic procedure and provide pre- and postcare related to diagnostic procedure • Administer the drugs • Provide health education • Perform basic resuscitation	• Taking pediactric history • Perform physical examination and assessment of children • Administration of oral, IM, and IV, medicine/fluid • Calculation of fluid requirements • Prepare different strengths of IV fluids • Apply restraints • Administer O_2 inhalation by different methods • Feed children by katori (bowl) and spoon, paladai, etc. • Collect specimens for common investigations • Assist with common diagnostic procedure • Teach mothers/parents on balance diet for child of different age group • Oral rehydration therapy • Feeding and weaning • Play therapy • Check vital signs • Give enema • Insert suppositories	• Give care to assigned pediatric patients • Nursing care plan – 1 • Case study or presentation – 1 • Health talk – 1	• Assess performance with rating scale • Assess each skill with checklist • Evaluation of nursing care plan, case study, health talk, case presentation • Completion of activity record
Pediatric surgery ward	3 weeks	• Recognize different pediatric surgical condition • Provide pre- and postoperative care to children with common pediatric conditions/ malformation	• Do bowel wash • Care for ostomies: ▪ Colostomy irrigation ▪ Ureterostomy ▪ Gastrostomy ▪ Enterostomy • Urinay catheterization and drainage	• Give care to three assigned pediatric surgical patients • Nursing care plan – 1	• Assess performance with rating scale • Assess each skill with checklist

Contd…

Areas	Duration	Objectives	Skill	Assignment	Assessment Methods
		• Counsel and educate parents	• Feeding ▪ Nasogastric ▪ Gastrostomy ▪ Jejunostomy • Care of surgical wound dressing • Suture removal	• Case study or presentation – 1	• Evaluation of nursing care plan, case study, case presentation • Completion of activity record
Pediatric OPD/ immunization room/well baby clinic/ adolescent clinic	4 weeks	• Perform assessment of children, health development and anthropometric • Perform immunization • Give health education/nutritonal education	• Assessment of children • Health assessment • Developmental assessment • Anthropometric assessment • Immunization • Health/nutritional education	• Health assessment of child • Health talk – 1 • IMNCI module	• Assess performance with rating scale • Completion of activity record • Assessment of the health talk

Contents

Preface v
Acknowledgments vii
Syllabus xiii

1. Clinical Procedures
- Neonatal Assessment 3
- Neonatal Resuscitation 5
- Anthropometric Assessment 8
- History Collection 12
- General Calculations Related to Children 15

2. Growth and Developmental Study
- Newborn 16
- Infant 21
- Toddler (1–3 Years) 26
- Preschooler (3–6 Years) 32
- School Going Child (6–12 Years) 38
- Adolescent (12–16 Years) 43

3. Nursing Care Plan
- Evaluation Criteria for Nursing Care Plan – 1 48
- Nursing Care Plan – 1 49
- Evaluation Criteria for Nursing Care Plan – 2 63
- Nursing Care Plan – 2 64
- Evaluation Criteria for Nursing Care Plan – 3 78
- Nursing Care Plan – 3 79

4. Case Study
- Evaluation Criteria for Case Study – 1 93
- Case Study – 1 94
- Evaluation Criteria for Case Study – 2 119
- Case Study – 2 120

5. Health Talk
- Evaluation Criteria for Health Talk – 1 145
- Content for Health Talk 146
- Evaluation Criteria for Health Talk – 2 148
- Content for Health Talk 149

6. Nanda-Approved Nursing Diagnoses 2021–23 143

STUDENT'S PROFILE

Paste Your
Passport Size
Photo

Name of the Student: ____________________

Reg. No./Enroll No.: ____________________

Course/Year: ____________________

Subject: ____________________

Batch: ____________________

University: ____________________

Name of the Institute: ____________________

Address of the Institute: ____________________

Signature of the Student | **Signature of the Subject Coordinator** | **Signature of the Principal**

Signature of the Internal Examiner | **Signature of the External Examiner**

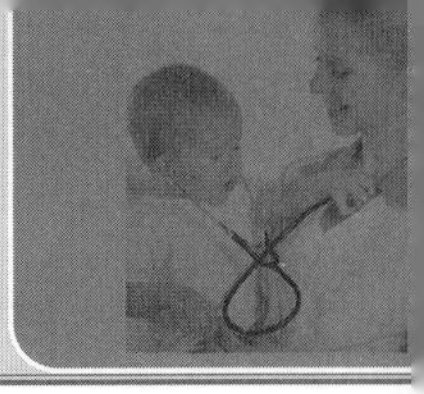

NEONATAL ASSESSMENT

Neonatal period starts at birth till 28 days following birth. Neonatal life is a period of transition from life in utero to adjustment to the external environment where he is exposed to varied conditions. The baby during this stage is still vulnerable due to the limited metabolic capacity and immaturity in organs.

According to period of gestation they are classified as:

- **Preterm:** When the gestational period is <37 weeks
- **Term:** When the gestational age is >37 weeks till 42 weeks
- **Post-term:** Gestational age >42 weeks

According to weight:

- **Low birth weight (LBW):** Birthweight <2,500 g
- **Very low birth weight (VLBW):** Birthweight <1,500 g
- **Extremely low birth weight (ELBW):** Birthweight <1000 g

According to weight for gestational age:

- **Small for gestation (SGA):** Weight <10th percentile
- **Appropriate for gestational age (AGA):** Weight from 10th to 90th percentile
- **Large for gestational age (LGA):** Weight >90th percentile.

ASSESSMENT OF GESTATIONAL AGE: THE NEW BALLARD SCORE

Gestational age of the newborn sometimes needs assessment. It is best performed within 48 hours of birth so that prematurity or postmaturity can be assessed and appropriate measures and care can be taken to avoid complications. It is applicable for newborns of gestational age 26–44 weeks. Each parameter score ranges from 2 to 5. The tool has two major components—neuromuscular maturity with 6 criteria and physical maturity, also with 6 criteria. The limitation of this scoring system is in case ELBW babies for which deviation is found to be for over 2 weeks.

NEUROMUSCULAR MATURITY

	–1	0	1	2	3	4	5
Posture	—						—
Square window (wrist)	>90°	90°	60°	45°	30°	0°	—
Arm recoil	—	180°	140°–180°	110°–140°	90°–110°	<90°	—
Popliteal angle	180°	160°	140°	120°	100°	90°	<90°
Scarf sign							—
Heel to ear maneuver							—

PHYSICAL MATURITY

Skin	Sticky, friable, transparent	Gelatinous red, translucent	Smooth, pink; visible veins	Superficial peeling and/or rash; few veins	Cracking, pale areas; rare veins	Parchment, deep cracking; no vessels	Leathery, racked wrinkled
Lanugo	None	Sparse	Abundant	Thinning	Bald areas	Mostly bald	Maturity rating
Plantar surface	Heel-toe 40–50 mm –1 <40 mm; –2	> 50 mm, no crease	Faint red marks	Anterior transverse crease only	Creases anterior ⅔	Creases over entire sole	
Breast	Imperceptible	Barely perceptible	Flat areola, no bud	Stippled areola, 1–2 mm bud	Raised areola 3–4 mm bud	Full areola 5–1 mm bud	
Eye/Ear	Lids fused loosely –1 tightly –2	Lids open; pinna flat; stays folded	Slightly curved pinna; soft; slow recoil	Well curved pinna; soft but ready recoil	Formed and firm, instant recoil	Thick cartilage, ear stiff	
Genitals (male)	Scrotum flat, smooth	Scrotum empty, faint rugae	Testes in upper canal, rare rugae	Testes descending few rugae	Testes down, good rugae	Testes pendulous deep rugae	
Genitals (female)	Clitoris prominent labia flat	Clitoris prominent small labia flat	Clitoris prominent enlarging minora	Major and minora equally prominent	Majora large, minora small	Majora cover clitoris and minora	

MATURITY RATING

Score	Weeks
–10	20
–5	22
0	24
5	26
10	28
15	30
20	32
25	34
30	36
35	38
40	40
45	42
50	44

Gestations by Dates

	Weeks

Birth date	Hour	
		am
		pm

APGAR	1 minute	5 minutes

Scoring

Gestational age by maturity rating	Weeks
Time of examination	Date______am Hour______pm
Age during examination	_________Hours

NEONATAL RESUSCITATION

PEDIATRIC RESUSCITATION ALGORITHM

Pediatric Basic Life Support Alogrith for Healthcare Providers Single Rescuer

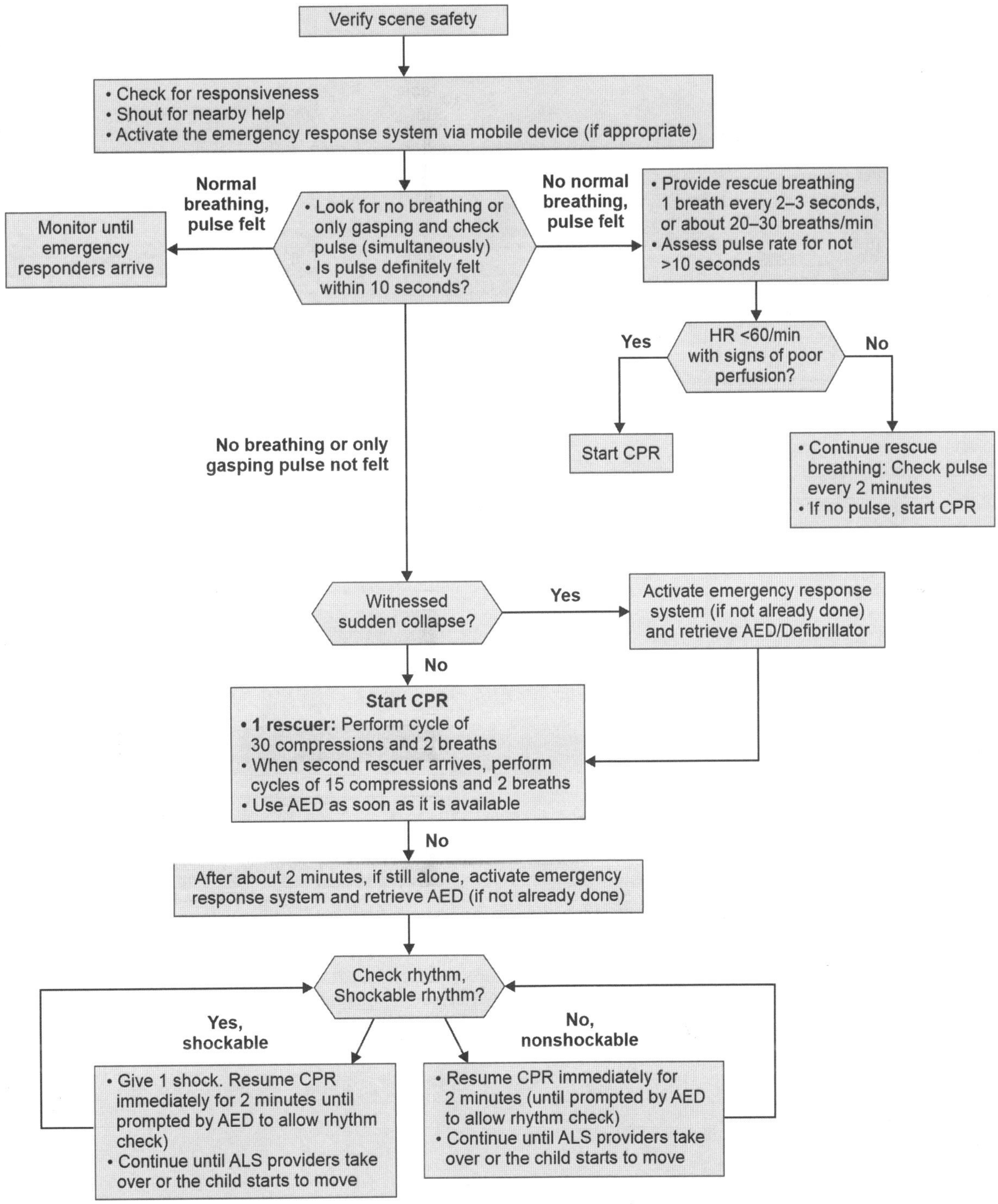

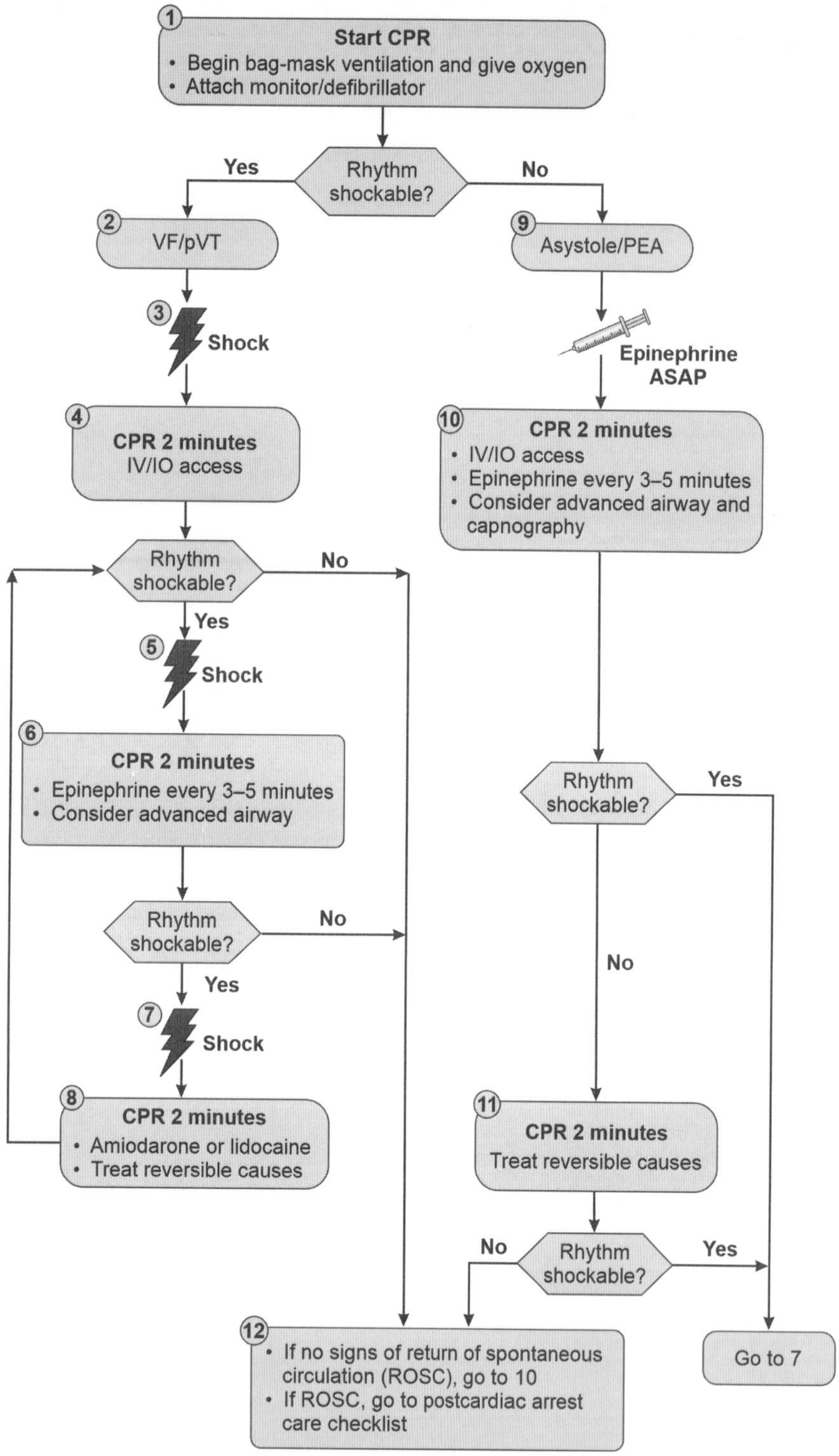

CPR quality

- Push hard (≥1/3 of anteroposterior diameter of chest) and fast (100–120/min) and allow complete chest recoil
- Minimize interruptions in compressions
- Change compressor every 2 minutes, or sooner if fatigued
- If no advanced airway, 15:2 compression-ventilation ratio
- If advanced airway, provide continuous compressions and give a breath every 2–3 seconds

Shock energy for defibrillation

- First shock 2 J/kg
- Second shock 4 J/kg
- Subsequent shocks ≥ 4 J/kg, maximum 10 J/kg or adult dose

Drug therapy

- Epinephrine IV/IO dose:
  0.01 mg/kg (0.1 mL/kg of the 0.1 mg/mL concentration).
  Max. dose 1 mg.
  Repeat every 3–5 minutes.
  If no IV/IO access, may give endotracheal dose: 0.1 mg/kg (0.1 mL/kg of the 1 mg/mL concentration)
- Amiodarone IV/IO dose: 5 mg/kg bolus during cardiac arrest. May repeat up to 3 total doses for refractory VF/pulseless VT
  or
  Lidocaine IV/IO dose:
  Initial: 1 mg/kg loading dose

Advanced airway

- Endotracheal intubation or supraglottic advanced airway
- Waveform capnography or capnometry to confirm and monitor ET tube placement

Reversible causes

- Hypovolemia
- Hypoxia
- Hydrogen ion (acidosis)
- Hypoglycemia
- Hypo-/hyperkalemia
- Hypothermia
- Tension pneumothorax
- Tamponade, cardiac
- Toxins
- Thrombosis, pulmonary
- Thrombosis, coronary

Source: American Heart Association Guidelines 2020

APGAR SCORING

First examination is done at birth during which Apgar scoring is done to assess a baby's condition after birth and adaptability at birth. It was described by Dr Virginia Apgar (anesthesiologist) in 1952. It has breathing, heart rate, muscle tone, reflexes and color as its main components. It is done at 1 minute, 5 minutes and rarely at 10 minutes to see how well the baby can adapt outside the mother's womb.

Criteria/score	0	1	2
Breathing	Absent	Slow, gasping	Crying
Heart rate	Absent	Up to 100	More than 100
Musclet one	Flaccid	In between	Fully flexed
Reflexes	Nil	Grimace	Cough, sneeze, cry
Color	Blue/pale	Peripheral cyanosis	Pink

Score from 7 to 10 is normal, 4 to 6 fairly low (need O_2) 3 and <3 — critically low (need artificial ventilation)

- Second examination is done within few hours of birth for:
  - Successful adaptation to extrauterine life
  - Screening for congenital anomalies [like tracheoesophageal fistula (TEF), spina bifida, diaphragmatic hernia, annorectal anomalies, etc.]
  - For conducting anthropometric assessment.

ANTHROPOMETRIC ASSESSMENT

Anthropometry is used to assess physical growth in children using noninvasive method to assess body size, weight, body proportion, etc., and is universally applicable. It includes measurement of weight, height/length, arm span, head circumference, chest circumference, abdominal circumference, body proportion; mid upper arm circumference and skin fold thickness.

1. **Weight:** It is the most important indicator of growth and nutritional status and is recommended by Indian Academy of Pediatrics (IAP) for use to assess the severity of malnutrition.

   Pattern of increase:

   - A term baby weights between 2.9 and 3.2 kg (40 weeks). Thereafter, baby loses 10% of birth weight during first three days and is regained within 10 days.

Age	Weight gain in grams/day
0–3 months	30
3–6 months	20
6–9 months	15
9–12 months	12
1–3 years	1.0

   - The infants doubles his weight by 5 months, triples by one year and quadruples by 2 years.
   - After 2 years weight gain till adolescence is 2–2.5 kg/year.
   - Weight gain is also rapid during puberty

   The following are the formulas to calculate the expected weight according to age.

Weight	Formula
3–12 months	Weight = (age in months + 9)/2
1–6 years	Weight = 2 (age in years) + 8
7–12 years	Weight = [7 (age in years) – 5]/2

2. **Height/length:** For children who can stand steadily (above 2 years) standing height is measured, with the shoes removed, using a stadiometer (ideally) or a stature meter with head in frankfort plane and occiput, back of knees, buttocks and heels touching the flat surface.

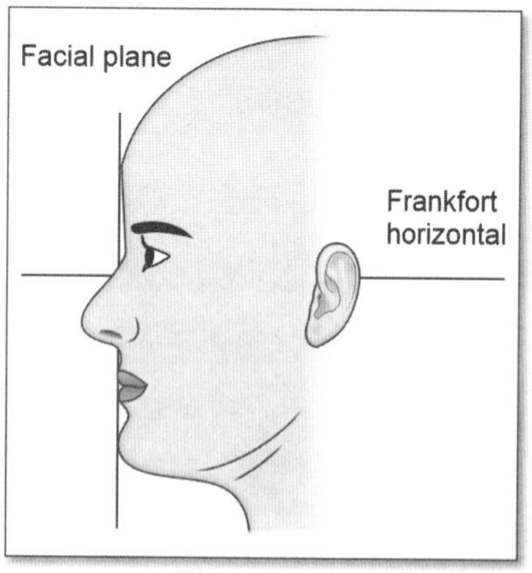

Figure 1: Frankfort plane

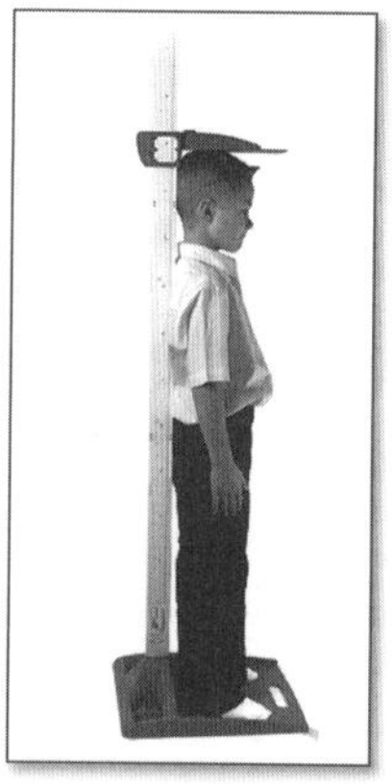

Figure 2: Stadiometer

For infants and children below 2 years an infantometer is used to measure the length of the child. The legs are straightened using pressure on the knees. The foot board is brought in contact with the child's feet and the length is measured.

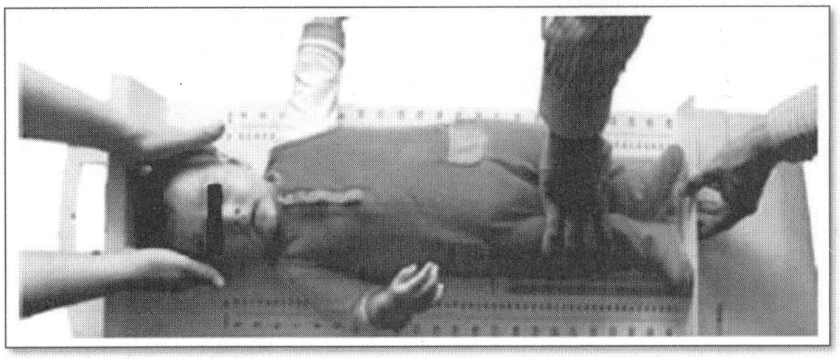

Figure 3: Infantometer

An average Indian child has a length of about 50 cm which becomes 75 cm by 1 year and 90 cm by 2 years.

The formula to calculate expected height for children (2–12 years) is:

Height = (age in years × 6) + 77

3. **Head circumference:** It is measured using a nonstretchable tape. It is measured over biparietal eminence and above supraorbital ridges. It about 35 cm at birth and increase by 10–12 cm during first year of life, thereafter increases by 2 cm in second year and then 0.5 cm/year till 8 years of age.

Age	Head growth per month (in cm)
0–3 months	2.0
3–6 months	1.0
6–9 months	0.5
9-12 months	0.5
1–3 years	0.2

4. **Chest circumference:** Itis measured over the nipples and midway between inhalation and exhalation using a nonstretchable tape. This parameter in 2–3 cm less than head circumference at birth, becomes equal around 1 year and then is more than head circumference.
5. **Mid upper arm circumference:** It is 9–11 cm at birth and is around 16 cm by 1 year than after the circumference increases very slowly (0.25 cm/year) so is considered constant. It can be taken as age-independent criteria to assess malnutrition and can be used to assess malnutrition from 6 to 60 months of age. A child having a mid arm circumference <12.5 cm is considered severe malnutrition. It is measured with the arm in the neutral position, the length from acromion to olecranon process is divided into three parts and is taken at the level of middle part.

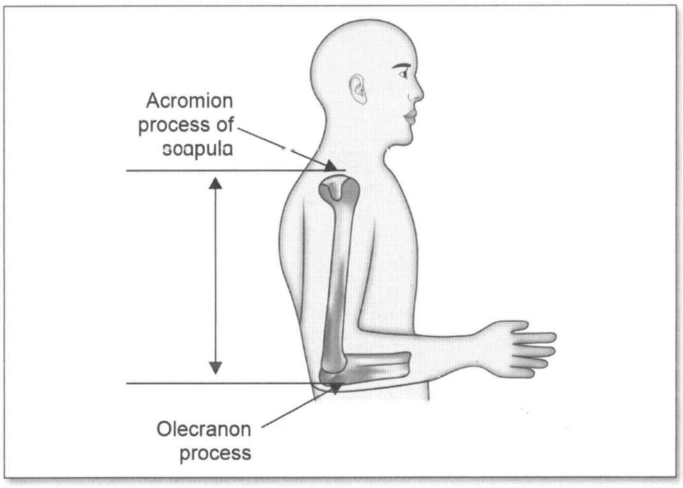

Figure 4: Mid upper arm circumference

A special tape called Shakir's tape is used, it has three zones —red, yellow and green corresponding to severity to malnutrition (normal (>13.5 cm), moderate (12.5–13.5 cm) and severe (<12.5 cm).

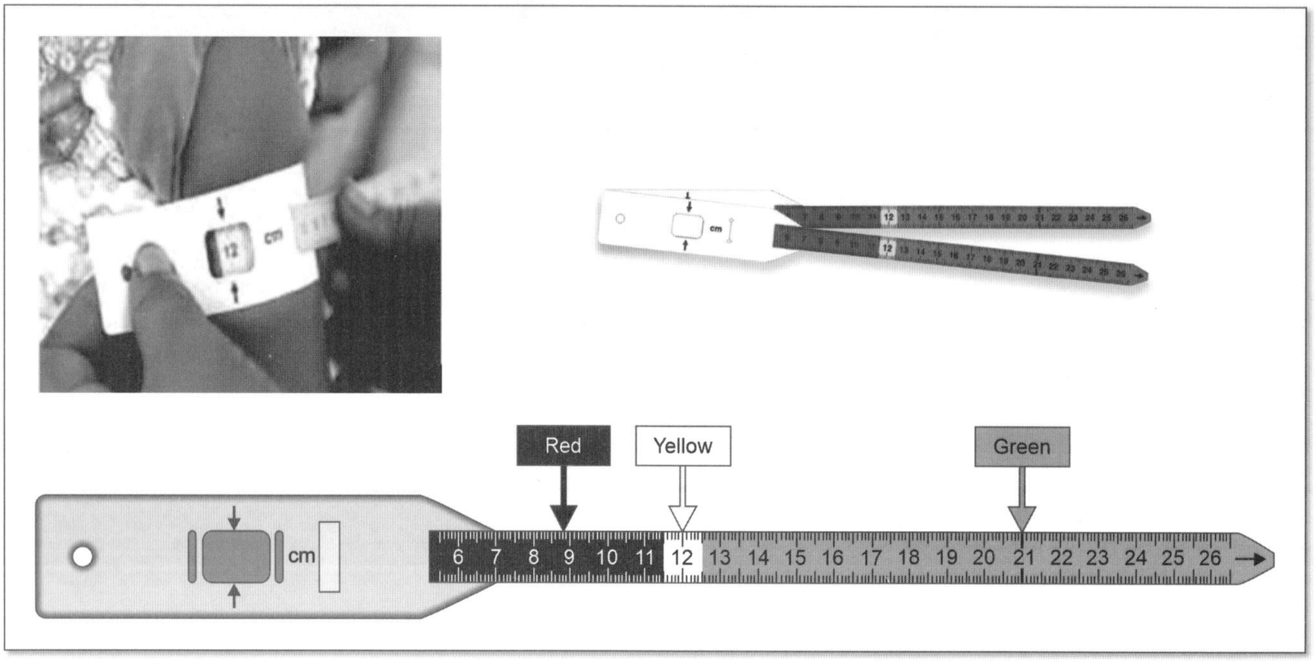

Figure 5: MUAC-Tape

6. **Arm span:** It is used sometimes as a measure to estimate height of children in condition when the child is not able to stand due to some musculoskeletal or neurological problem. It is taken as distance between the tip of middle finger of one hand and another when the arms are stretched at 90° to the body. It is less than height by 1–2 cm by the age of 10 years and then after is less than height by 3–5 cm.

INTERPRETATIONS

- When weight/age is less it is called underweight.
- When height/age is less than normal it is called stunting.
- When weight/height is less it is called wasting.
- A normal child usually follows the same percentile during his childhood.
- It mainly changes during sickness or adolescent stage.

According to **Indian Academy of Pediatrics (IAP)** Protein energy malnutrition can be identified using the following classification:

Grades of malnutrition	% age of expected weight/age
Grade I	71–80%
Grade II	61–70%
Grade III	51–60%
Grade IV	>50%
K	Denotes presence of edema

***Expected weight can be calculated as = Child's weight/ideal weight (value of 50th percentile/value calculated from the formula) × 100**

Example: A child is 3-year-old and weighs 13 kg, so we will first calculate his ideal or expected weight = 2 (age in years) + 8 = 2 (3) + 8, i.e., 14 kg

Now to assess malnutrition =13/14 × 100 = 92.8% (i.e., the child is not malnourished)

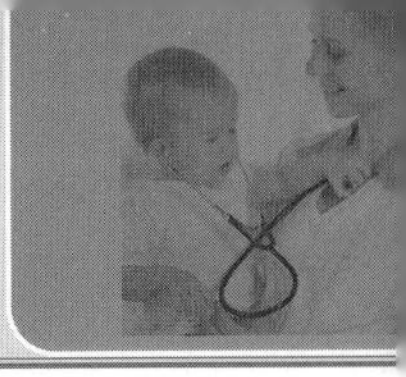

WHO CLASSIFICATION OF MALNUTRITION

Types of PEM	% of body weight compared to standard weight	Edema	Deficiency in weight for height
Kwashiorkor	80–60	+	+
Marasmic kwashiorkor	<6	+	++
Marasmus	<60	Nil	++
Nutritional dwarfism	<60	Nil	Nil
Underweight	80–60	Nil	Nil

HISTORY COLLECTION

OBTAINING HISTORY OF ILLNESS IN A CHILD

OBJECTIVES

- History taking is the first steps toward rapport building with the child and the family.
- It gives an idea about the nature and course of illness in the child and provides with the detail of clinical problems in the child.
- It also helps frame nursing diagnoses for the child.
- Helps nurse to plan care for the child based on the problems explained by the child or the family.

METHOD AND SEQUENCE OF HISTORY TAKING

- The procedure requires private and comfortable place for the child and parents, especially when collecting information from adolescents as they are privacy conscious.
- The nurse must identify the reliable source of information which at times may be other than parents.
- The nurse must know the language known to the parents for accurate comprehension of information.
- Open-ended questions must be asked to get parents version of illness.
- History must be obtained in a nonformal way and as a part of natural conversation. Avoid addition of own interpretation as it can change the meaning of what has been said.
- Unnecessary details, probing and judgments must be avoided.

SEQUENCE

History is obtained from present health condition to past health status.
- Chief complaints for which the child is hospitalized.
- Present health complaints which the child may have for some time.
- Past health conditions include a history of any medical/surgical problem or any infection.
- Family history is important as some conditions or disease run in families and may also be preventable to some extent. Common familial conditions are thalassemia, hemophilia, metabolic disorders, etc.
- Personal details of birth, development, immunization and feeding, etc.

Chief complaints with which the child was brought to the hospital are noted in chronological order in the order of their appearance and the duration or the episode (e.g., fever for 3 days, vomiting for 2 days (7 episodes). Only significant complaints are considered some complaint are associated with main symptom (e.g., bodyache, restlessness may occur due to fever).

Apart from main complaints the aggravating or suppressing factors are also enquired, associated signs and symptoms are also asked for (For example for foul smell, abdominal pain with diarrhea, fever and vomiting and varying degree of dehydration can also occur)

Present health condition—Conditions with a long course of illness are included in this section. The time of onset of illness (when did the problem start), course taken as abrupt onset, insidious (slow and gradual) onset, severity of present illness, diurnal variations in the symptoms and treatment taken so far and effectiveness of the treatment. A negative history is also taken to rule out involvement of other systems. This is done by assessing or reviewing the major signs and symptoms related to each system.

SYSTEM-WISE MAJOR SIGNS

General condition	Growth parameters such as height, weight, head and chest circumference, activity (normal, decreased, over activity), behavior (normal, shy, aggressive, outspoken, etc.) sleep and appetite
Respiratory system	Cough, dyspnea, stridor, retractions, asthma, etc.

Contd...

GI system	Nausea, vomiting, abdominal distension, decreased or increased bowel sounds, jaundice and worm infestations
Cardiovascular system	Cyanosis, cool clamy skin, pulses (apical peripheral), palpitations, blood pressure, heart sounds and edema
Nervous system	Seizures, altered consciousness, headache, macro/microcephaly, meningeal signs and vomiting
Genitourinary system	Delayed or precocious sexual characters, menarche pain discharge, burning micturition, oliguria, polyuria, and hematuria
Hematology	Anemia, fatigue, petechiae, ecchymosis, epistaxis, inherited blood disorders

Past health history: Previous episodes of illnesses and hospitalization are enquired. Any history of surgery, its cause, description of surgical procedure and occurrence of area specific problem (endemic problems). The treatment taken, medications, their intake, amount and schedule is also important to note. Compliance with the treatment is also important to note (e.g., tuberculosis has a low compliance).

PERSONAL HISTORY

Birth history includes antenatal, natal and family history:

- Antenatal period in an important phase as the baby is still developing and is affected by maternal health condition which is also a determinant of baby's health. Maternal history of diabetes, hypertension, etc., must be noted. History of antenatal checkups and findings of various tests are important.
- Natal history—gestational age at birth gives a picture of anticipated problems. Apgar score at birth, adverse event, birthweight, resuscitation need, ICU stay duration (if any) general health status are indicators of growth potential of child.
- **Family history** of illness is important as some disorders and illnesses have a genetic tendency and the family that shares the same environment,nutritionally, economically has an equal chance of having the same problems. Life style related problems like obesity, hypertension, diabetes, etc., and habits like smoking, drinking, drug abuse are also assessed. Current illness in the family has a bearing on the child especially if it is infectious.
- Making a pedigree chart is important to have an understanding of family and if possible a three generation chart must be prepared. The commonly used symbols in a pedigree chart are as follows:

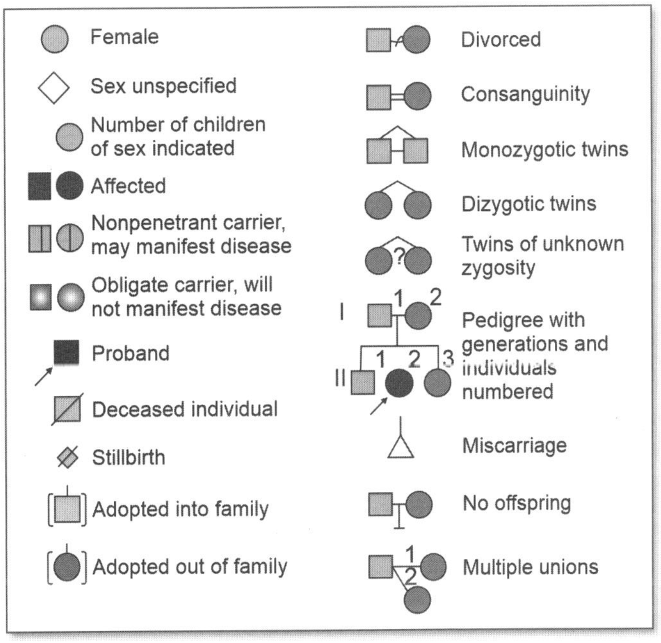

Figure 6: Pedigree chart

- **Developmental history:** Child developmental stage must match his age. Note danger signs related to age of achievement of milestones which might indicate developmental delay. DDST is a common tool used for developmental assessment.

IMMUNIZATION

Status must be completed and age and date of vaccine administration must be noted.
National immunization schedule recommends the following schedule of vaccines:

Vaccine	Timing	Dose	Route	Site
BCG	At birth or as early as possible till one year of age	0.1 mL (0.05 mL until 1 month of age)	Intradermal	Left upper arm
Hep. B	At birth or as early as possible till 24 hours	0.5 mL	Intramuscular	Anterolateral side of mid-thigh
OPV birth dose	At birth or as early as possible within 15 days of life	2 drops	Oral	Oral
OPV 1, 2 and 3	At 6 weeks, 10 weeks and 14 weeks	2 drops	Oral	Oral
fIPV	At 6 weeks and 14 weeks	0.1 mL	Intradermal two fractional dose	Intradermal: Right upper arm
PCV	At 6 weeks 14 weeks and booster 9 months	0.5 mL	Intramuscular	Anterolateral side of mid-thigh
Pentavalent 1, 2 and 3	At 6 weeks, 10 weeks and 14 weeks	0.5 mL	Intramuscular	Anterolateral side of mid-thigh
Rotavirus	At 6 weeks, 10 weeks and 14 weeks	5 drops	Oral	Oral
Measles rubella 1st dose	9–12 months (give up to 5 years if not received at 9–12 months)	0.5 mL	Subcutaneous	Right upper arm
Vitamin A 1st dose	At 9 months with measles	1 mL (1 lakh units)	Oral	Oral
DPT 1st booster	16–24 months	0.5 mL	Intra muscular	Anterolateral side of mid-thigh
OPV booster	16–24 months	2 drops	Oral	Oral
Measles and rubella 2nd dose	16–24 months	0.5 mL	Subcutaneous	Right upper arm
Vitamin 2nd – 9th dose	16 months with DPT/OPV booster then one dose every 6 months upto 5 years	2 mL (2 lakh units)	Oral	Oral
DPT 2nd booster	5–6 years	0.5 mL	Intramuscular	Ventrogluteal area
Td	10 years and 16 years	0.5 mL	Intramuscular	Ventrogluteal area

- After 9 years—HPV (up to 14 years 2 doses 1 and 6 months apart, 14 years onward 3 doses 0, 2 and 6 months apart).
- IPV is recommended to immunocompromised children and a part of postpolio eradication policy).
- Breastfeeding does not interfere with development of immunity.
- A number of vaccines can be given in combination at different sites, however there must be gap of 4 weeks between two live vaccines.

Socioeconomic status includes parent education, occupation and family income. Per capita income determination helps plan treatment and use of other modalities that can be afforded by the family. It also includes housing, drinking water source, hobbies, food habits, cooking methods used.

ANALYZING HISTORY

History collection helps the nurse reach the following:
- Nature of illness (duration, course and treatment).
- Organ systems involved in illness.
- Probable cause, aggravating and precipitating factors of illness.
- Possible complications and prognosis.

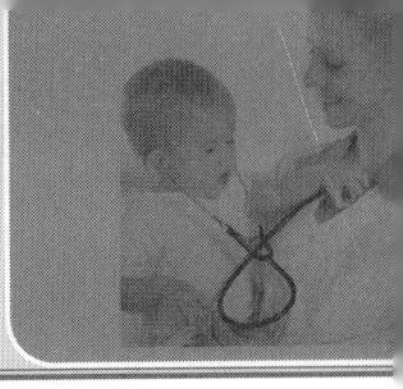

GENERAL CALCULATIONS RELATED TO CHILDREN

1. CALORIC REQUIREMENTS

Body weight	Calories requirement
0–10 kg	100 kcal/kg/day
10–20 kg	1000 kcal + 50 kcal/kg/day (for each kg)
>20 kg	1500 kcal + 20 kcal/kg (for each kg)

2. FLUID REQUIREMENTS

Body weight	Fluid	Infusion rate
>10 kg	100 mL/kg/day	4 mL/kg/hr
10–20 kg	1000 + 50 mL/for each kg above 10/day × (weight – 10)	40 mL/hr + 2 mL/kg/hr × (weight – 10)
20–30 kg	1000 + 500 + 20 mL/for each kg above 20/day	60 mL/hr + 1 mL/kg/hr × (weight – 20)

3. DRUG CALCULATION

- **Clark's rule:** Child dose = adult dose × (weight of child (in lbs) ÷ 150)
- **Young's rule:** Child dose = adult dose × (age of child ÷ [age of child +12])

Basic Rule for Calculation

Amount to be given = desired dose ÷ dose in hand × amount available

For calculating drop rate/min = volume to be infused (in mL) ÷ time in minutes × drop factor

For a pediatric drip set the drop factor to 60 (16 for macro drip set)

GROWTH AND DEVELOPMENTAL STUDY

NEWBORN

1. Name of the Baby ______________________________
2. Sex ______________________________
3. Mother's Name ______________________________
4. Father's Name ______________________________
5. Ward/Area ______________________________
6. Date of Birth ______________________________
7. Gestational Age ______________________________
8. Mode of Delivery ______________________________
9. Diagnosis (Medical/Surgical) ______________________________

   Date of Surgery (if any) ______________________________
10. Informant ______________________________
11. Date of Assessment ______________________________

PHYSICAL ASSESSMENT

Assessment criteria	Present/absent in baby	Remarks
Vitals • Heart rate: 100–120 bpm		
• Respiration-abdominal/thoracoabdominal: 40–60/min		
• Temperature: 36.5°–37.5°C		
• Blood pressure: 80/50 mm Hg		
General appearance • Attitude–flexion		
• Good muscle tone		
• Pink color		
• Vigorous		
• Vernix caseosa in body folds (neck, axilla, groin)		
Head • Normal symmetry		
• Caput succedaneum		
• Cephalohematoma		
• Craniotabes/craniosynostosis		
Hair • Normal distribution		
• Sparse		
• Silky, lustrous		
• Fine, wooly/fuzzy		
Circumference (33–35 cm) • Anterior fontanelle (2.5 × 4 cm)		
• Posterior fontanelle (0.5 × 0.5 cm)		
• Flat/depressed/bulging		
Eyes • Slant (mongoloid/antimongoloid)		
• Hypo/hypertelorism		
• Eyelids (swollen/puffy)		
• Sclera (white/yellow)		
• Blinking reflex		
• Corneal reflex		
• Eye movements		

Contd...

Assessment criteria	Present/absent in baby	Remarks
Nose • Nasal flaring		
• Discharge		
• Nasal patency		
• Nasal polyps/mass		
Ears • Alignment with helix of ear (lowset)		
• Discharge		
• Pre auricular tag/sinus		
Lips and Mouth • Lip color (pink/cyanosed)		
• Cleft lip		
• Oral mucosa color (pink/cyanosed/yellow)		
• Cleft palate		
• Palatal arch (normal/high)		
• Natal teeth		
• Ankyloglossia (tongue tie)		
• Macro/microglossia		
• Ebstein pearls		
Neck • Normal range of motion		
• Birth injury (torticollis)		
• Short/broad		
• Webbed neck		
Chest • Eupnea		
• Chest in drawing/retractions		
• Pectuscarinatum/exacavatum		
• Nipples alignment		
• Chest circumference (1.5–2 cm less than head circumference)		
• Breast bud size		
• Swollen/discharge from breast buds (Witch's milk)		
• Protruding chest (CDH) in relation to abdomen		
• Normal S_1 S_2 (4 thintercostal space midclavicular line)		

Contd...

Assessment criteria	Present/absent in baby	Remarks
Abdomen • Shape (protruding/scaphoid) distension/visible blood vessels abdominal girth		
• Umbilical stump (dry/swelling/discharge)		
• Cord (dry/shed off)		
Genitalia • Urination Frequency		
Male • Penis (approx. 2.5 cm)		
• Urethral meatus (central/dorsal/ventral)		
• Scrotum (pendulous/small/dark pigmented/lightly pigmented/rugae/testes descended/undescended)		
Female • Clitoris (hypertrophied)		
• Labia minor covered/exposed (by labia majora) Pseudomenstruation		
• Urethral meatus-(normal)		
Anal area • Anal opening patent/stenosed/imperforate		
• Ectopic/anterior anus		
• Meconium passage—(normal/fistula)		
• Stool passing—(frequency)		
Extremities • Hip dislocation—(ortolani/barlow maneuver)		
• Poly/syn/clino/oligodactyly		
• Hand creases—present		
• Simian crease		
• Sole creases—present		
• Club foot (talipes/calcaneus/varus/valgus)		
Back • Normal C-shaped curve		
• Any abnormal curvature (cervical/thoracic/lumbar/lateral) Tuft of hair (lumbosacral area)		
• Mongolian spots		

NEONATAL/PRIMITIVE REFLEXES

Reflex	Elicitation	Response	Age of disappearance	Findings in baby
Rooting	Stroke the corner of mouth or cheek with finger or nipple	The head turns toward the stimulus	3–4 months	
Sucking	Stroking the lowerlip	Sucking action and tongue protrudes out	3–4 months	
Blinking	Flash of light on eyes or puff of air	Blinking action	Remains	
Grasping	Touching the palm with finger or pen	Baby holds the pen or finger tightly	Starts disappearing around 3 months	
Moro's (startle)	Sudden loud noise (sleeping baby) or movement If awake, elevate the baby's head with one hand and drop for 1 cm supporting the neck	Baby gets startled extension of arms and legs, then adduction	3–4 months	
Stepping	Hold the baby up right with feet touching the surface	Baby makes walking motion	3–4 months	
Babinski	Stroke the base of toe	Fanning of the fingers and dorsiflexion of the toe	9–10 months	
Gag reflex	Excess food in the mouth	Clears throat and prevents choking	Remains	
Asymmetric Tonic neck reflex (fencing)	Turn the face toward one side	Ipsilateral extension of arm and hands contralateral flexion	3–4 months	
Doll's eye	Turn the baby's face slowly toward one side	Normally eyes do not move	3–4 months	
Extrusion	The baby extrudes any material placed over anterior tongue	Tongue pushes outward on stroking the tongue with object	3–4 months	
Parachute	Hold baby in ventral suspension and move forward rapidly	Arm sex tend to prevent falling (like a parachute)	3–4 months	

Teacher's Signature

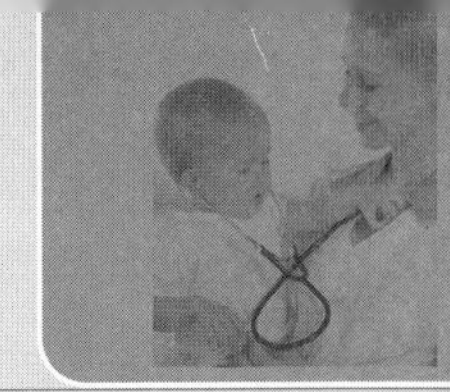

GROWTH AND DEVELOPMENTAL STUDY

INFANT

1. Name of the Baby ____________________

2. Sex ____________________

3. Mother's Name ____________________

4. Father's Name ____________________

5. Ward/Area ____________________

6. Date of Birth ____________________

7. Diagnosis (Medical/Surgical) ____________________

   Date of Surgery (if any) ____________________

8. Informant ____________________

9. Date of Assessment ____________________

GROWTH PARAMETERS

Criteria	Normal values/formula	Findings/interpretation
Vitals	**Temperature:** 36.5°–37°C	
	Pulse: 80–120 bpm	
	Respiration: 20–40 breaths/min	
	Blood pressure: 80/50 mm Hg	
Anthropometric values	**Head circumference:** 45–47 cm	
	Head circumference=Chest circumference (from 6 months till 2 years)	
	Mid upper arm circumference: 16 cm	
	Weight: (age in months + 9)/2	
	Doubles birth weight at 5 months	
	Triples birth weight at 1 year	
	Height: Approx. 75 cm	
	Malnutrition grade (if any) = age of child/ideal weight × 100	

Table: Developmental milestones

Age/domain	Gross motor development	Observation
0–4 weeks	• Sucks reflexively • Visually tracks tomidline • Lifts head when held up right	
3–4 months	• Prone: Lifts head • Momentarily: Rolls from stomach to back • Pulls to sit without head lag	
5–6 months	• Grasps rattle • Reaches for objects • Inspects objects with hands, eyes, and mouth	
6–9 months	• Creeps • Sits without support • Pulls to stand or cruise furniture	
9–12 Months	• Crawls on all fours • Attains sitting position unaided • Stands momentarily • Takes first steps	

Age/domain	Fine motor	Observation
6–9 months	• Transfers objects from one hand to another hand • Bangs with spoon • Shakes bell	
9–12 Months	**9–12 months** • Holds, bites and chews a cracker • Beats two spoons together • Begins to use index finger to point and poke	

Age/domain	Personal/social	Observation
0–4 weeks	**0–8 weeks** • Gazes at faces (birth) • Smiles responsively • Uses vocalization to interact socially	
3–4 months	• Distinguishes primary care givers from others • Smiles readily at most people • Plays alone with contentment	

Contd...

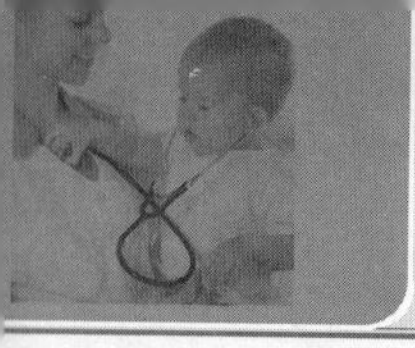

Age/domain	Personal/social	Observation
6–9 months	• Stranger/separation anxiety begins • Seeks attention; wants to be picked up and held • Plays peek aboo • Pats own mirror image • Chews and bites toys • Begin to respond to own name	
9–12 Months	• Social with family, shy with strangers • Begins to show sense of humor • Becomes aware of emotions of others	

Age/domain	Language and cognition	Observation
3–4 months	• Babbles and coos, squeals and gurgles(by 3 months) • Anticipates food with vocalization • Laughs	
6–9 months	• Smiles and vocalizes to own mirror image • Says 'ma-ma,' 'dada' • Imitates playful sounds • Turns head to being called	
9–12 Months	• Repeats performances that are laughed at • Plays peekaboo • Waves bye bye • Calls mama, dada	

DEVELOPMENTAL ASPECTS–AS PER HISTORY OBTAINED

Domain	Milestones	Observation/action
Moral	• Self-centered • No judgment of right or wrong	
Spiritual **Undifferentiated/primal faith**	• The baby has faith in the care of others and significant others	
Intellectual reflexive stage (0–2 months)	• Simple reflex activity such as grasping, and sucking	
Primary circular reactions (2–4 months)	• Reflexive behaviors such as opening and closing fingers repetitively, sucking thumb to indicate need for feed or sleep	
Secondary circular reactions (4–8 months)	• Repetition of actions to produce interesting consequences using a rattle to produce sound.	
Coordination of secondary reactions (8–12 months)	• Actions are intentional such as reaching behind a screen to obtain a hidden object.	

Teacher's Signature

GROWTH AND DEVELOPMENTAL STUDY

TODDLER (1–3 YEARS)

1. Name of the Child ______________________

2. Sex ______________________

3. Mother's Name ______________________

4. Father's Name ______________________

5. Ward/Area ______________________

6. Date of Birth ______________________

7. Diagnosis (Medical/Surgical) ______________________

   Date of Surgery (if any) ______________________

8. Informant ______________________

9. Date of Assessment ______________________

GROWTH PARAMETERS

Criteria	Normal values/formula	Findings/interpretation
Vitals	**Temperature:** 36.5°–37°C	
	Pulse: 70–100 bpm	
	Respiration: 20–30 breaths/min	
	Blood pressure: 85/55 mm Hg	
	Else use formula • Systolic **BP** = 90 + (age in years × 2) • Diastolic **BP** = 55 + (age in years × 2)	
Anthropometric values	Head circumference—48, 49 and 50 cm at 2 years, 3 years and 4 years respectively	
	Chest circumference > head circumference	
	Mid upper arm circumference = 16 cm	
	Weight: 2 (age in years) + 8 or 2 years: 12 kg, 3 years: 15 kg, 4 years: 16 kg	
	Height: 2 years — 90 cm, 3 years — 95 cm, 4 years —100 cm	
	Malnutrition grade (if any) = weight of child/ideal weight × 100	

Table: Developmental milestones

Age/domain	Gross motor development	Observation
12–18 months	• Walks alone or with one hand held • Broad-based gait • Climbs up on furniture • Walks up stairs with hand held • Can run stiffly	
18–24 months	• Runs stiffly • Pushes and pulls large objects • Carries large toys • Seats self in small chair	
24–30 months	• Jumps in place • Walks up and down steps, both feet on each step • Walks backward • Runs well • Opens door	
30–36 months	• Builds tower of 6–8 cubes • Completes 3-piece form board.	

Age/domain	Fine motor	Observation
12–18 months	• Builds tower of 2–4 cubes • Scribbles spontaneously • Imitates vertical line • Feeds from cup • Puts raisin or pellet in mouth • Turns book pages, 2–3 at a time	
18–24 months	• Builds tower of 4–6 cubes • Tries to fold paper imitatively • Turns pages singly • Turns knobs • Imitates vertical line • Takes off shoes	
24–30 months	• Holds pencil with thumb and fore fingers • Zips and unzips self • Builds tower of 6–8 cubes • Tower of 7 cubes • Copies vertical line, • Imitates horizontal line • Turns pages of books singly • Uses buttons, zippers, buckles	
30–36 months	• Turns book pages singly • Holds pencil with thumb and forefingers.	

Contd...

Age/domain	Personal/social	Observation
12–18 months	• Plays simple ball game • Finger feeding • Indicates wants by poiting at objects • Hugs parents • Symbolic play • Feeds independently • Gives toy to adult on request • Imitates adult activities • Interested in strangers	
18–24 months	• Helps dress and undress self • May indicate wet or soiled diapers • Asks for food and drink by vocalizing and gesturing • Uses spoon with little spilling • Wants to have care giver near by all the time • Plays alone or beside other children • Follows simple requests • Shows temper tantrums	
24–30 months	• Drinks from cup without spilling • Begins toilet training • Dry by day • Listens to stories, uses picture books • Initiates own play activities • Does not like change in routine • Cannot wait or delay gratification.	
30–36 months	• Begins playing 'with', as opposed to 'next to others' • Names or points to self in photos • Likes praise • Has auditory fears (noises, thunderstorm) • Washes hands, brushes teeth • Plays games in parallel with other children	

Age/domain	Language and cognition	Observation
12–18 months	• Communicates by gesture • Vocalizes more than crying for attention • Understands word 'no' • Shakes head to indicate no • Says 2–3 'words' other than 'ma-ma' or 'da-da.'	
	• Vocabulary of 10–15 words • Points and vocalizes to indicate wants.	

Contd...

Age/domain	Language and cognition	Observation
18–24 months	• Points to pictures in books • Points to one body part • Has vocabulary of 20 words—mostly nouns • Enjoys simple stories • Speaks in 2 word sentences (e.g., he gone)	
24–30 months	• Often calls self by first name • Speaks 50 or more words • Has vocabulary of 300 words • Uses phrases and 3–4 words sentences • Points to 4 body part	
30–36 months	• Verbalizes toilet needs • Uses plural • Increases use of verbs • Begins using adjectives and prepositions • Has vocabulary of 900–1,000 words (36 months) • Gives full name when asked	

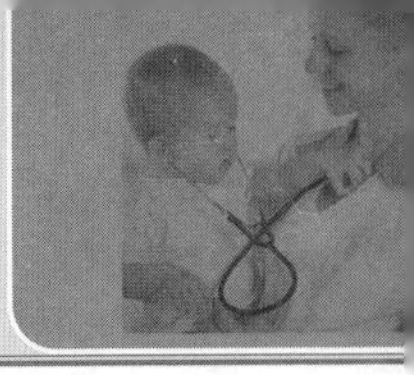

DEVELOPMENT ASPECTS–AS PER HISTORY OBTAINED

Domain	Milestones	Observation/action
Moral (preconventional morality)	• Punishment obedience—certain action should not be done to avoid punishment. For example, we must not steal to avoid going to jail • Good is what I like	
Spiritual	• Faith related to magical thinking • Performs religions actions without conceptual development	
Intellectual (preoperational 2–7 years, preconceptual 2–4 years)	• Mental representation of objects and identification • Egocentric thinking, logic and reasoning not developed	

Teacher's Signature

GROWTH AND DEVELOPMENT

PRESCHOOLER (3–6 YEARS)

1. Name of the Baby ______________________

2. Sex ______________________

3. Mother's Name ______________________

4. Father's Name ______________________

5. Ward/Area ______________________

6. Date of Birth ______________________

7. Diagnosis (Medical/Surgical) ______________________

   Date of Surgery (if any) ______________________

8. Informant ______________________

9. Date of Assessment ______________________

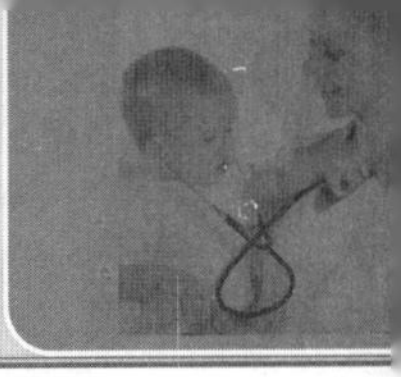

GROWTH PARAMETERS

Criteria	Normal values/formula	Findings/interpretation
Vitals	**Temperature:** 36.5° – 37°C	
	Pulse: • 1–5 years = 70–100 bpm • 5–10 years = 60–80 bpm	
	Respiration: 20–30 breaths/min	
	Blood pressure: 85/55 mm Hg **Else use formula** • Systolic BP = 90 + (age in years × 2) • Diastolic BP = 55 + (age in years × 2)	
Anthropometric values	**Head circumference** • Boys: 37–47 cm • Girls: 35.8–46 cm	
	Chest circumference > head circumference	
	Mid upper arm circumference: 16 cm	
	Weight: • Boys: 11.4–26.7 cm • Girls: 11–27.3 cm **Height:** • Boys: 89–125 cm • Girls: 88–124.8 cm	
	Malnutrition grade (if any) = age of child/ideal weight × 100	

Table: Developmental milestones

Age/domain	Gross motor development	Observation
3 years	• Gallops • Catches large ball, arms flexed • Hops on one foot (3 times) • Turns some results • Shows lack of coordination stumbling, falling	
4 years	• Runs at varying speeds • Hops on one foot (4–9 times) • Balances on one foot (8 seconds) • Throws ball over hand • Handless stairs with alternating feet using rails	
5 years	• Balances on one foot • Skips smoothly • Uses roller skates • Rides bicycle with training wheels • Balances on tip toes	
6 years	• Constantly active • Shows smooth and coordinated movement • Stands on one foot, eyes closed • Has good balance and rhythm • Bounces ball with good control	
Age/domain	**Fine motor**	**Observation**
3 years	• Copies circle • Imitates cross • Builds tower of 10 cubes • Spontaneously draws • Imitates snipping with scissors	
4 years	• Copies cross and square • Established hand dominance • 'Writes' on page at random • Draws person with arms and legs directly from head	
5 years	• Handedness firmly established • Colors within lines • Copies circle, square,and triangle • Draws within small areas • Ties knot in string after demonstration	
6 years	• Ties own shoes • Makes simple, recognizable drawings	

Contd...

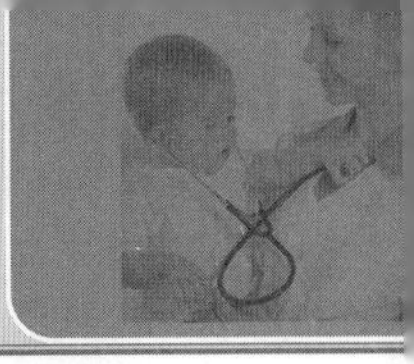

Age/domain	Personal/social	Observation
3 years	• Is ready to conform to spoken word • Begins to take turns • Plays simple group games • Toilets self during the day • Shows fear (visual fears, heights, loss of parent, etc.) • May have imaginary play mates • Plays with others • Shares upon request	
4 years	• May be physically aggressive • Has night mares • Separates from mother easily • Washes face, brushes teeth and dresses self • Uses bathroom unassisted	
5 years	• Enjoys small group cooperative play—often noisy • Listens and participates in group activity • Enjoys competitive exercise games • Respects peers and their property	
6 years	• Poor ability to modulate feelings • Shows jealousy of others • Very competitive • Often insists on having own way • Goes to bed unassisted • Often takes small things from others and claims they found them • Begins to distinguish right and left onself	

Age/domain	Language and cognition	Observation
3 years	**Receptive language** • Follows two unrelated commands • Has concept of 2 or 3 • Identifies 2–3 colors • Listens attentively to short stories • Chooses objects that are hard/soft, heavy/light, big/little **Expressive language** • Uses sentences • Answers yes/no questions • Repeats nursery rhymes • Counts 2–3 items • Has vocabulary of 1,500 words • Tells age using fingers • Understands past versus present • Shows curiosity; asks endless questions • Matches colors (2 or 3) • Answers sensibly to “Why do we have stoves?” etc. • Tells a simple story	

Contd...

Age/domain	Language and cognition	Observation
4 years	**Receptive language** • Follows 3-stage commands • Listens eagerly to stories • Follows directions with prepositions (e.g., 'above,' 'under') **Expressive language** • Uses all parts of speech correctly • Has vocabulary of 2,000-plus words • Uses color names • Asks many questions (e.g., why, what, how)	
5 years	**Receptive language** • Listens briefly to what others say • Understands 6,000 words • Categorize words • Guesses object by attribute or use of clues **Expressive language** • Has vocabulary of 2,500 words • Acts out stories • Learns left from right • Matches 10–12 colors • Writing mostly in capitals • Recognizes first name • Recognizes several or all • Writes 1–10 poorly • Adds and subtracts using 5 fingers	
6 years	**Receptive language** • Uses picture dictionary • Knows category labels • Defines and explains words **Expressive language** • Identifies likeness and differences between objects • Gives category labels • Likes to use big words **Cognitive development** • Names all colors • Knows what number comes after • Understands quantity up to 10 • Identifies similarities and differences among pictures • School Milestones • Matches words • Rereads books many times • Writes first and last name. • Subtracts numbers within 5 • Uses simple measurement	

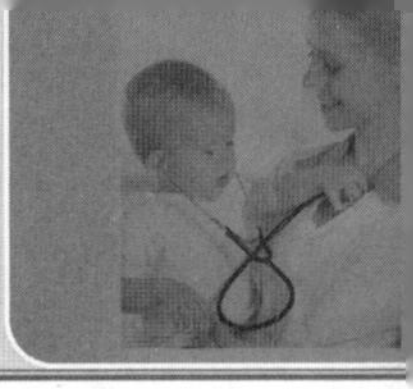

OTHER DEVELOPMENT ASPECTS

Domain	Milestones	Observation/action
Moral (preconventional morality, individual, instrumentation and exchange state)	• Understand others needs and desires • Want rewards for being good (why should I be good with others?)	
Spiritual	• Faith related to magical thinking • Performs religions actions without conceptual development	
Intellectual (preoperational 2–7 years, preconceptual 2–4 years, 4–7 years intuitive thoughts)	• Mental representation of objects and identification • Ego centric thinking, logic and reasoning not developed • Develops an idea of conservation of mass, number and area	

Teacher's Signature

GROWTH AND DEVELOPMENT

SCHOOL GOING CHILD (6–12 YEARS)

1. Name of the Child ______________________________

2. Sex ______________________________

3. Mother's Name ______________________________

4. Father's Name ______________________________

5. Ward/Area ______________________________

6. Date of Birth ______________________________

7. Diagnosis (Medical/Surgical) ______________________________

   Date of Surgery (if any) ______________________________

8. Informant ______________________________

9. Date of Assessment ______________________________

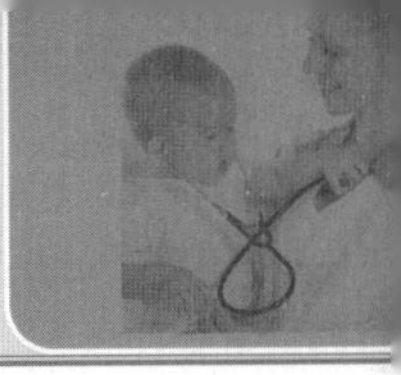

GROWTH PARAMETER

Criteria	Normal values/formula	Findings/interpretation
Vitals	**Temperature:** 36.5°–37°C	
	Pulse: • 6–10 years = 70–110 bpm • 11–14 years = 60–105 bpm	
	Respiration: • 6–10 years = 15–30 minutes • 11–14 years = 12–20 minutes **Blood pressure:** 6–13 years Systolic: 85–120; Diastolic: 55–80	
Anthropometric values	**Weight** = 27–46 kg 1–6 years weight = 2 (age in years) + 8 7–12 years weight = [7 (age in years) – 5]/2	
	Height = 125–164 cm (2–12 years) Height = (age in years × 6) + 77	
	Malnutrition grade (if any) = Age of child/ideal weight × 100	

Table: Developmental milestones

Age/domain	Gross motor and physical development	Observation
6–9 years	• Rides bicycle • Holds pencil, toothbrush, and tools easily • Enjoys exercise of both large and small muscles • Becomes interested in competitive sports—social aspects of sports • Shows poor posture (e.g., head close to work)	
Age/domain	**Fine motor**	**Observation**
6–9 years	• Has well-developed small muscles • Has well-developed hand-eye coordination • Draws triangle in good proportion • Copies vertical and horizontal diamonds	
Age/domain	**Personal/social**	**Observation**
6–9 years	• Shows independence in routines • Becomes quiet when angry • Better control of voice and temper • Anxious to please others; sensitive to praise and blame • Has not learned to lose games • Concerned about right and wrong • Criticizes opposite sex • Makes same sex child as special friend	
Age/domain	**Language and cognition**	**Observation**
6–9 years	• Speaks fluently • Understands cause 0 effect relationships • Recites days of week and months of year • Internal sense of time emerges • Shows increasing reading vocabulary • Learns to solve addition and subtraction combinations • Cursive writing • Addition substractions, multiplication	
Age/domain	**Physical development**	**Observation**
9–10 years	• Girls and boys even in size and sexual maturity (early in 10th year) • Girls' bodies undergo light softening and rounding at 10th year • Shows little awareness of fatigue • Strongly refuses bathing • Loves outdoor exercise play (e.g., baseball, skating, jumping rope, running)	

Contd...

Age/domain	Physical development	Observation
10–12 years	• Pubic hair pigmented, curled • Axillary hair begins after pubic hair • Height growth spurt • Breast development continues • Prepubescent physical development • Beginning growth of testes, scrotum, and penis	
Age/domain	**Personal/social**	**Observation**
9–10 years	• Boys show friendship with physical expression (e.g., punch, wrestle) • Girls show friendship with gossiping, hand-holding • Enjoys sharing secrets and discussing mysteries with friends • Believes friends over parents	
10–12 years	• Yells and calls names • Rarely cries except with hurt feelings • Tends to have sincere, trusting, and physically affectionate relationship with mother • Tends to have positive, adoring, admiring relationship with father • Has abrupt mood and behavior swings • Females highly concerned with body image, physical changes • Increasingly interested in peers and peer culture • Changes in friends are common	
Age/domain	**Cognitive**	**Observation**
9–10 years	• Interest in reading varies. • Repeats dirty, jokes to parent, but often does not understand them • Interested in his or her future a parent and how he or she will treat own child	
10–12 years	• Rarely interested in keeping a diary • Mostly interested in material possessions, • Enjoys memorizing. • Prefers oral to written work in school • Shows short interest span—needs frequent shift of activity in school • Decreased interest in movies and television	

OTHER DEVELOPMENT ASPECTS

Domain	Milestones	Observation/action
Moral (conventional morality, interpersonal conformity, group focused) and law and order (society focused)	• Wants to do right things and to be called good boy (good and bad boy concept) • Learns trust, loyalty and gratitude • Feels internal compulsion for abiding societal norms • Respect for authority	
Spiritual (Synthetic-conventional faith)	• Faith is based on the feelings of right or wrong. Feel related to groups. Take responsibility for their action • Related freedom with accountability	
Intellectual (preoperational 2–7 years, preconceptual 2–4 years, 4–7 years intuitive thoughts)	• Develop concept of compensation, identity and reversibility • Learn classification of things	

Teacher's Signature

GROWTH AND DEVELOPMENT

ADOLESCENT (12–16 YEARS)

1. Name of the Child ______________________________

2. Sex ______________________________

3. Mother's Name ______________________________

4. Father's Name ______________________________

5. Ward/Area ______________________________

6. Date of Birth ______________________________

7. Diagnosis (Medical/Surgical) ______________________________

   Date of Surgery (if any) ______________________________

8. Informant ______________________________

9. Date of Assessment ______________________________

GROWTH PARAMETERS

Criteria	Normal values/formula	Findings/interpretation
Vitals	**Temperature:** 36.5°–37°C	
	Pulse: 15–20 years (60–100 bpm)	
	Respiration: 15–20 years (12–30 bpm)	
	Blood pressure: 13–18 years Systolic: 95–140; Diastolic: 60–90 mm Hg	
Anthropometric values	**Weight:** 45–60 kg	
	Height: 162–187 cm (boys); 164–175 cm (girls)	
	Malnutrition grade (if any) = age of child/ideal weight × 100	

Table: Developmental milestones

Age/domain	Physical development	Observation
Early adolescence: 11–13 years	**Females** • Pubic hair pigmented, curled • Axillary hair begins after pubic hair • Height growth spurt • Breast development continues • Labia enlarged • Menstruation begins **Males** • Prepubescent physical development • Beginning growth of testes, scrotum, and penis • Downy pubic hair • Consistent height growth	
Mid adolescence: 13–15 years	**Females** • Pubic hair fully developed • Axillary hair in moderate quantity • Continued breast growth • Menstruation established • Decelerating height velocity • Ovulation(fertility) • Moderate muscle growth and increase in motor skills **Males** • Pubic hair pigmented and curled • Axillary hair begins after pubic hair • Penis, testes, and scrotum continue to grow • Height/growth spurt • Seminal emissions but sterile • Voice deepens as larynx enlarges • Mustache hair appear	
Late adolescence: 15–16 years	**Females** • Full development of breasts and axillary hair • Decelerated height growth (ceases at 16 years ± 13 months) **Males** • Facial and body hair • Pubic and axillary hair denser • Voice deepens	

Contd...

Age/domain	Personal/social	Observation
Early adolescence: 11–13 years	• Anxious about peer acceptance • Concerned with self-identity • Egocentric • Abrupt mood and behavior swings • Girls highly concerned with body image, physical changes • Changes in friends are common • Same -sex relationships develop • Have concerns, anxiety with opposite sex • Strong needs for achievement and recognition of accomplishment	
Mid adolescence: 13–15 years	• Increasingly independent from family • Females become more comfortable with body image and changes • Males highly concerned with body image and changes as puberty begins • Shows increase in relationships with opposite sex; however same-sex relationship continues to dominate • Reliance on peer relationships • May experiment with drugs • Concerned with achievement, experiences • Continues to be interested in appearance, music, and other elements of peer culture	
Late adolescence: 15–16 years	• Increase in anxiety and avoidance behaviors • Concerned and interested in movement toward independence; generally not prepared emotionally or logistically for complete emancipation	

Age/domain	Cognitive	Observation
Early adolescence: 11–13 years	• Begins to move from concrete toward abstract thinking (reasoning) • Increasingly interested in ideas, values, social issues • Interested in music and personal appearance—especially girls • Increasing conflicts with family • Places strong value on family and parents	
Mid adolescence: 13–15 years	• Shows fully developed abstract thought and can apply in more situations • Anxiety, major distractions interfere with abstract thinking • Continued interest in ideas, ideals, values, social issues	
Late adolescence: 15–16 years	• Shows well-established abstract thinking • Makes applications to own current and future situations and to broader issues (e.g., social concerns, academic studies)	

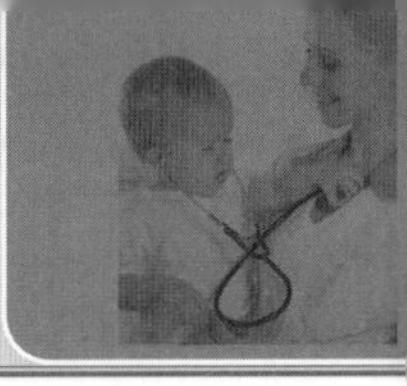

OTHER DEVELOPMENT ASPECTS

Domain	Milestones	Observation/action
Moral (postconventional, social contract and individual rights, universal/ethical principles stage)	• Child learns variability of norms in different cultures and societies • Obeys laws and principles which are in line with universal benefit	
Spiritual (individuative-reflective faith)	• Makes personally meaningful of commitments • Develops an inner value system, own values and beliefs may question earlier beliefs	
Intellectual (formal operations)	• Develops abstract thinking • Apply logic to real life situations	

Teacher's Signature

EVALUATION CRITERIA FOR NURSING CARE PLAN – 1

Name of Patient ____________________

Ward/Area ____________________

Diagnosis ____________________

Registration No. ____________________

Criteria	Max. marks	Marks obtained
Identification data	2	
History collection	3	
Problem assessment	5	
Nursing diagnosis framed	5	
Care planned according to priority	3	
Care implemented	2	
Evaluation	5	
Total score	**25**	

Teacher's Signature

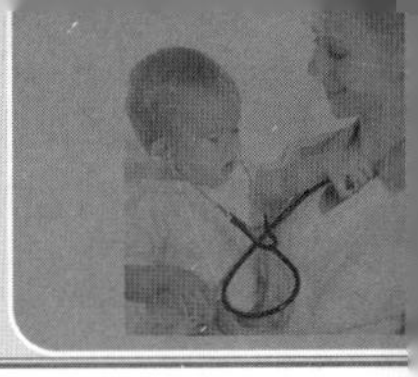

NURSING CARE PLAN – 1

1. Name of the Child ______________________________

2. Sex ______________________________

3. Mother's Name ______________________________

4. Father's Name ______________________________

5. Ward/Area/Bed No. ______________________________

6. Date of Birth/Age ______________________________

7. Diagnosis (Medical/Surgical) ______________________________

   Date of Surgery (if any) ______________________________

8. Informant ______________________________

9. Date of Assessment ______________________________

10. Period of Care From ____________________ Till ____________________

HISTORY

Chief Complaints on Admission

Present Health History (Medical/Surgical)

Past Health History (Medical/Surgical)

Birth History (Antenatal/Intranatal/Postnatal)

Family History of Illness

Pedigree Chart

Socioeconomic Background

Food Habits–Vegetarian/Nonvegetarian/Ovo-vegetarian

Likes and Dislikes in Food Items

Allergy

Elimination Pattern

Development According to Age (Assess Milestones)

Play Activities

Growth Assessment

1. Height
2. Weight
3. Head circumference
4. Chest circumference
5. Mid upper arm circumference

Inference

Malnutrition = Actual weight/Expected weight × 100 = Grade (if any) I/II/III/IV.

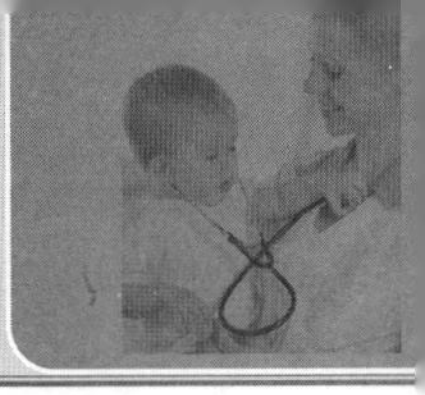

Immunization History

Age	Vaccine	Given in child/date
At birth	BCG OPV Hep-B	
6 weeks	OPV Rotavac 1 Pentavac 1 (DPT + Hep. B + HiB)	
10 weeks	OPV Rotavac 1 Pentavac 1 (DPT + Hep. B + HiB)	
14 weeks	OPV Rotavac 1 Pentavac 1 (DPT + Hep. B + HiB) IPV	
9 months	Measles/MR 1, booster PCV	
16–24 months	Measles/MR 2 OPV DPT booster	
5–6 years	DPT booster	
10 and 16 years	Td	

PHYSICAL ASSESSMENT

Physical features	Present in child	Any other deviation
General appearance		
• Level of consciousness	Conscious/unconscious/lethargic/stuporous	
• Posture	Normal/kyphosis/scoliosis/lordotic/guarding	
• Body built	Normal/under/overnourished/thin built	
• Facial expression	Apathy/apprehensive/depressed/normal	
• Gait	Steady/unsteady/limp	
• Ambulation	Bedridden/ambulating	
• Skin color	Pallor/cyanosis/flushed	
Vitals		
• Heart rate/pulse	--------bpm	
• Temperature	------------°C	
• Respiration	------------/min	
• Blood pressure	-----/--------mm Hg	
Head		
• Size and shape	Normal/shape	
• Circumference	Normocephalic/macro/microcephaly	
• Hair texture and distribution	Lustrous/coarse/sparse/normal distribution	
• Scalp	Dandruff/infestation (pediculosis)/infection	
• Fontanels: Anterior and posterior	Closed/open/enlarged/flat/depressed/bulging	
Eyes		
• Lids and lashes	Swelling/hemorrhage/lesion	
• Distance (placement)	Hypo/hypertelorism present/absent	
• Discharge movements	Normal/restricted gauge	
• Conjunctiva	Hemorrhage/inflammation	
• Vision (aquity/color)	Normal acquity/color blindness	
Ears		
• Low-set	Present/absent	
• Discharge	Present/absent	
• Preauricular tag/sinus	Present/absent	
• Microtia/macrotia/anotia	Present/absent	
• Hearing	Normal/abnormal	
Nose		
• Flaring	Present/absent	
• Discharge	Present/absent	
• Abnormality	Depressed nasal bridge/deviated nasal septum	

Contd...

Physical features	Present in child	Any other deviation
Mouth		
• Lips—color/cleft	Pink/cyanosis/cleft	
• Palate—cleft/arch	Cleft/high arch	
• Tongue—coated, thrush	Present/absent	
• Abnormality	Macro/microglossia/drooling/mouth wide open	
• Oral mucosa	Pink/cyanosis/yellow	
• Dentition	Complete/incomplete/malocclusion/caries	
• Throat-inflammation	Present/absent	
Neck and Chest		
• **Neck**		
▪ Short/webbed	Present/absent	
▪ Lymphadenopathy	Present/absent	
▪ Birth injury/torticollis	Present/absent	
▪ Range of motion	Normal/restricted	
▪ Thyroid gland	Enlarged/normal	
▪ Tracheal deviation	Present/absent if present (R/L)	
• **Chest**		
▪ Shape and sternum	Normal/pectus carinatum/excavatum	
▪ Symmetry and movement	Equal bilateral/unequal	
▪ Work of breathing	Normal/eupnea/increased (use of accessory muscles)	
▪ Any abnormalities	Any mass/precordial bulge/heave	
▪ Circumference		
▪ Air entry	Equal bilateral/decreased (R/L)	
▪ Breath sounds	Normal/abnormal (wheeze/crackles)	
▪ Percussion	Dullness/resonance	
▪ Heart sounds	Normal S_1-S_2/murmurs/gallops/third sound	
▪ Axillary lymph nodes	Enlarged/normal	
Abdomen		
• Shape	Normal/asymmetry	
• Bowel sounds	Audible/inaudible	
• Fluid	Present/absent	
• Distension/tenderness	Present/absent	
• Girth	Hepatomegaly/splenomegaly	
• Organomegaly (liver/spleen)	Any other mass	
• Abnormality	Present/absent	

Contd...

Physical features	Present in child	Any other deviation
Perineum and Genitalia		
Male genitalia		
• Urinary meatus/stream	Central/dorsal/ventral/normal stream	
• Scrotum	Normal, pigmented/swelling	
• Testes	Descended/undescended	
• Any abnormality	Hydrocele/hernia	
Female genitalia		
• Labia minora and majora	Normal/abnormal	
• Urination	Normal/abnormal (burning)	
• Any infection	Present/absent	
Rectum and anus	Normal/ectopic/anterior	
• Anal position	Normal/abnormal	
• Patency/imperforation	Normal/abnormal	
• Elimination/stool pattern		
• Any deviation		
Extremities		
Hands and feet		
• Number of digits	Normal/poly/syn/oligo/dactyly	
• Nails	Pitted/spoon shaped/splinter hemorrhage	
• Clubbing	Present/absent	
• Creases	Simian crease/normal	
Back		
• Curvature	Normal/kyphosis/scoliosis/lordosis	
• Any tuft of hair	Present/absent	
• Pigmentation	Red rash/Mongolian spots	
• Any deviation		
Reflexes		
• Corneal		
• Pupillary		
• Abdominal		
• Biceps		
• Triceps		
• Brachioradialis		
• Knee jerk		
• Ankle jerk		
• Cremasteric (male)		
• Any other		
Impression (problems assessed)		

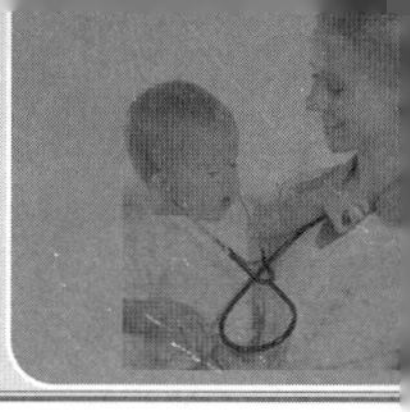

Nursing Diagnosis (Based on Problems Assessed)

1. ____________________
2. ____________________
3. ____________________
4. ____________________
5. ____________________
6. ____________________
7. ____________________
8. ____________________
9. ____________________
10. ____________________

Treatment Given

Physician Recommendations (Related to Care and Interventions)

____

____

____

____

Medicines and Fluids

Name (salt name)	Dose and route	Side effects	Nursing responsibility

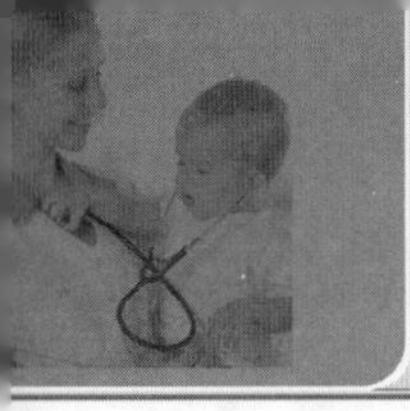

Diagnostic Tests

Test name	Findings	Remarks

Short-Term Goals

1. ______
2. ______
3. ______
4. ______
5. ______
6. ______
7. ______
8. ______
9. ______
10. ______

Long-Term Goals

1. ______
2. ______
3. ______
4. ______
5. ______
6. ______
7. ______
8. ______
9. ______
10. ______

Date/time	Nursing diagnosis	Goal	Intervention planned	Care given	Evaluation
Day 1 Subjective data					
Objective data					

Date/time	Nursing diagnosis	Goal	Intervention planned	Care given	Evaluation
Day 2 **Subjective data**					
Objective data					

Date/time	Nursing diagnosis	Goal	Intervention planned	Care given	Evaluation
Day 3 Subjective data					
Objective data					

Date/time	Nursing diagnosis	Goal	Intervention planned	Care given	Evaluation
Day 4 **Subjective data**					
Objective data					

Teacher's Signature

EVALUATION CRITERIA FOR NURSING CARE PLAN – 2

Name of Patient ______________________________

Ward/Area ______________________________

Diagnosis ______________________________

Registration No. ______________________________

Criteria	Max. marks	Marks obtained
Identification data	2	
History collection	3	
Problem assessment	5	
Nursing diagnosis framed	5	
Care planned according to priority	3	
Care implemented	2	
Evaluation	5	
Total score	**25**	

Teacher's Signature

NURSING CARE PLAN – 2

1. Name of the Child ______________________________

2. Sex ______________________________

3. Mother's Name ______________________________

4. Father's Name ______________________________

5. Ward/Area/Bed No. ______________________________

6. Date of Birth/Age ______________________________

7. Diagnosis (Medical/Surgical) ______________________________

   Date of Surgery (if any) ______________________________

8. Informant ______________________________

9. Date of Assessment ______________________________

10. Period of Care From ____________________ Till ____________________

HISTORY

Chief Complaints on Admission

____

____

____

____

Present Health History (Medical/Surgical)

____

____

____

____

Past Health History (Medical/Surgical)

____

____

____

____

Birth History (Antenatal/Intranatal/Postnatal)

____

____

____

____

Family History of Illness

____

____

____

____

Pedigree Chart

Socioeconomic Background

Food Habits–Vegetarian/Nonvegetarian/Ovo-vegetarian

Likes and Dislikes in Food Items

Allergy

Elimination Pattern

Development According to Age (Assess Milestones)

Play Activities

Growth Assessment

1. **Height** ______________________
2. **Weight** ______________________
3. **Head circumference** ______________________
4. **Chest circumference** ______________________
5. **Mid upper arm circumference** ______________________

Inference ______________________

Malnutrition = Actual weight/Expected weight × 100 = Grade (if any) I/II/III/IV.

Immunization History

Age	Vaccine	Given in child/date
At birth	BCG OPV Hep. B	
6 weeks	OPV Rotavac 1 Pentavac 1 (DPT + Hep. B + HiB)	
10 weeks	OPV Rotavac 1 Pentavac 1 (DPT + Hep. B + HiB)	
14 weeks	OPV Rotavac 1 Pentavac 1 (DPT + Hep. B + HiB) IPV	
9 months	Measles/MR 1, booster PCV	
16–24 months	Measles/MR 2 OPV DPT booster	
5–6 years	DPT booster	
10 and 16 years	Td	

PHYSICAL ASSESSMENT

Physical features	Present in child	Any other deviation
General appearance		
• Level of consciousness	Conscious/unconscious/lethargic/stuporous	
• Posture	Normal/kyphosis/scoliosis/lordotic/guarding	
• Body built	Normal/under/over nourished/thin built	
• Facial expression	Apathy/apprehensive/depressed/normal	
• Gait	Steady/unsteady/limp	
• Ambulation	Bedridden/ambulating	
• Skin color	Pallor/cyanosis/flushed	
Vitals		
• Heart rate/pulse	--------bpm	
• Temperature	------------°C	
• Respiration	------------/min	
• Blood pressure	-----/--------mm Hg	
Head		
• Size and shape	Normal/shape	
• Circumference	Normocephalic/macro/microcephalic	
• Hair texture and distribution	Lustrous/coarse/sparse/normal distribution	
• Scalp	Dandruff/infestation (pediculosis)/infection	
• Fontanels: Anterior and posterior	Closed/open/enlarged/flat/depressed/bulging	
Eyes		
• Lids and lashes	Swelling/hemorrhage/lesion	
• Distance (placement)	Hypo/hypertelorism	
• Discharge movements conjunctiva	Present/absent Normal/restricted gauge	
• Vision (aquity/color)	Hemorrhage/inflammation Normal acquity/color blindness	
Ears		
• Low-set	Present/absent	
• Discharge	Present/absent	
• Preauricular tag/sinus	Present/absent	
• Microtia/macrotia/anotia	Present/absent	
• Hearing	Normal/abnormal	
Nose		
• Flaring	Present/absent	
• Discharge	Present/absent	
• Abnormality	Depressed nasal bridge/deviated nasal septum	

Contd...

Physical features	Present in child	Any other deviation
Mouth		
• Lips—color/cleft	Pink/cyanosis/cleft	
• Palate—cleft/arch	Cleft/high arch	
• Tongue—coated, thrush	Present/absent	
• Abnormality	Macro/microglossia/drooling/mouth wide open	
• Oral mucosa	Pink/cyanosis/yellow	
• Dentition	Complete/incomplete/malocclusion/caries	
• Throat—inflammation	Present/absent	
Neck and Chest		
• **Neck**		
■ Short/webbed	Present/absent	
■ Lymphadenopathy	Present/absent	
■ Birth injury/torticollis	Present/absent	
■ Range of motion	Normal/restricted	
■ Thyroid gland	Enlarged/normal	
■ Tracheal deviation	Present/absent if present (R/L)	
• **Chest**		
■ Shape and sternum	Normal/pectus carinatum/excavatum	
■ Symmetry and movement	Equal bilateral/unequal	
■ Work of breathing	Normal/eupnea/increased (use of accessory muscles)	
■ Any abnormalities	Any mass/precordial bulge/heave	
■ Circumference		
■ Air entry	Equal bilateral/decreased (R/L)	
■ Breath sounds	Normal/abnormal (wheeze/crackles)	
■ Percussion	Dullness/resonance	
■ Heart sounds	Normal S_1, S_2/murmurs/gallops/third sound	
■ Axillary lymphnodes	Enlarged/normal	
Abdomen		
• Shape	Normal/asymmetry	
• Bowel sounds	Audible/inaudible	
• Fluid	Present/absent	
• Distension/tenderness	Present/absent	
• Girth	Hepatomegaly/splenomegaly	
• Organomegaly (liver/spleen)	Any other mass	
• Abnormality	Present/absent	

Contd...

Physical features	Present in child	Any other deviation
Perineum and Genitalia		
Male genitalia		
• Urinary meatus/stream	Central/dorsal/ventral/normal stream	
• Scrotum	Normal, pigmented/swelling	
• Testes	Descended/undescended	
• Any abnormality	Hydrocele/hernia	
Female genitalia		
• Labia minora and majora	Normal/abnormal	
• Urination	Normal/abnormal (burning)	
• Any infection	Present/absent	
Rectum and anus		
• Anal position		
• Patency/imperforation	Normal/ectopic/anterior	
• Elimination/stool pattern	Normal/abnormal	
• Any deviation	Normal/abnormal	
Extremities		
Hands and feet		
• Number of digits	Normal/poly/syn/oligodactyly	
• Nails	Pitted/spoon-shaped/splinter hemorrhage	
• Clubbing	Present/absent	
• Creases	Simian crease/normal	
Back		
• Curvature	Normal/kyphosis/scoliosis/lordosis	
• Any tuft of hair	Present/absent	
• Pigmentation	Red rash/Mongolian spots	
• Any deviation		
Reflexes		
• Corneal		
• Pupillary		
• Abdominal		
• Biceps		
• Triceps		
• Brachioradialis		
• Knee jerk		
• Ankle jerk		
• Cremasteric (male)		
• Any other		
Impression (problems assessed)		

Nursing Diagnosis (Based on Problems Assessed)

1. ___
2. ___
3. ___
4. ___
5. ___
6. ___
7. ___
8. ___
9. ___
10. ___

Treatment Given

Physician Recommendations (Related to Care and Interventions)

___

___

___

___

___

Medicines and Fluids

Name (salt name)	Dose and route	Side effects	Nursing responsibility

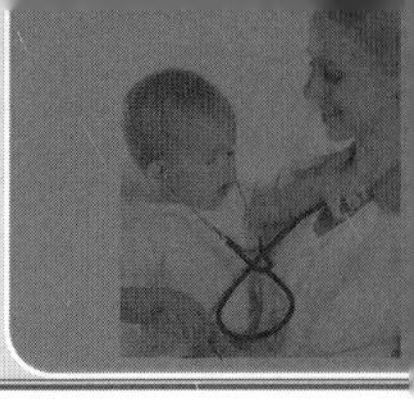

Diagnostic Tests

Test name	Findings	Remarks

Short-Term Goals

1. ______________________________
2. ______________________________
3. ______________________________
4. ______________________________
5. ______________________________
6. ______________________________
7. ______________________________
8. ______________________________
9. ______________________________
10. ______________________________

Long-Term Goals

1. ______________________________
2. ______________________________
3. ______________________________
4. ______________________________
5. ______________________________
6. ______________________________
7. ______________________________
8. ______________________________
9. ______________________________
10. ______________________________

Date/time	Nursing diagnosis	Goal	Intervention planned	Care given	Evaluation
Day 1 **Subjective data**					
Objective data					

Date/time	Nursing diagnosis	Goal	Intervention planned	Care given	Evaluation
Day 2 **Subjective data**					
Objective data					

Date/time	Nursing diagnosis	Goal	Intervention planned	Care given	Evaluation
Day 3 **Subjective data**					
Objective data					

Date/time	Nursing diagnosis	Goal	Intervention planned	Care given	Evaluation
Day 4 **Subjective data**					
Objective data					

Teacher's Signature

EVALUATION CRITERIA FOR NURSING CARE PLAN - 3

Name of Patient ____

Ward/Area ____

Diagnosis ____

Registration No. ____

Criteria	Max. marks	Marks obtained
Identification data	2	
History collection	3	
Problem assessment	5	
Nursing diagnosis framed	5	
Care planned according to priority	3	
Care implemented	2	
Evaluation	5	
Total score	**25**	

Teacher's Signature

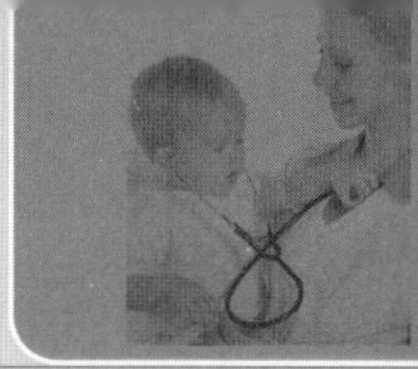

NURSING CARE PLAN – 3

1. Name of the Child ____________________

2. Sex ____________________

3. Mother's Name ____________________

4. Father's Name ____________________

5. Ward/Area/Bed No. ____________________

6. Date of Birth/Age ____________________

7. Diagnosis (Medical/Surgical) ____________________

   Date of Surgery (if any) ____________________

8. Informant ____________________

9. Date of Assessment ____________________

10. Period of Care From ____________________ Till ____________________

HISTORY

Chief Complaints on Admission

Present Health History (Medical/Surgical)

Past Health History (Medical/Surgical)

Birth History (Antenatal/Intranatal/Postnatal)

Family History of Illness

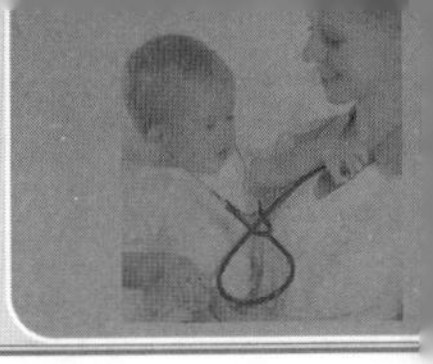

Pedigree Chart

Socioeconomic Background

Food Habits–Vegetarian/Nonvegetarian/Ovo-vegetarian

Likes and Dislikes in Food Items

Allergy

Elimination Pattern

____

____

____

____

____

Development According to Age (Assess Milestones)

____

____

____

____

____

Play Activities

____

____

____

____

____

Growth Assessment

1. **Height** ______________________________
2. **Weight** ______________________________
3. **Head circumference** ______________________________
4. **Chest circumference** ______________________________
5. **Mid upper arm circumference** ______________________________

Inference ______________________________

Malnutrition = Actual weight/Expected weight × 100 = Grade (if any) I/II/III/IV.

Immunization History

Age	Vaccine	Given in child/date
At birth	BCG OPV Hep.B	
6 weeks	OPV Rotavac 1 Pentavac 1 (DPT + Hep. B + HiB)	
10 weeks	OPV Rotavac 1 Pentavac 1 (DPT + Hep. B + HiB)	
14 weeks	OPV Rotavac 1 Pentavac 1 (DPT + Hep. B + HiB) IPV	
9 months	Measles/MR 1, booster PCV	
16–24 months	Measles/MR 2 OPV DPT booster	
5–6 years	DPT booster	
10 and 16 years	Td	

PHYSICAL ASSESSMENT

Physical features	Present in child	Any other deviation
General appearance		
• Level of consciousness	Conscious/unconscious/lethargic/stuporous	
• Posture	Normal/kyphosis/scoliosis/lordotic/guarding	
• Body built	Normal/under/overnourished/thin built	
• Facial expression	Apathy/apprehensive/depressed/normal	
• Gait	Steady/unsteady/limp	
• Ambulation	Bedridden/ambulating	
• Skin color	Pallor/cyanosis/flushed	
Vitals		
• Heart rate/pulse	--------bpm	
• Temperature	------------°C	
• Respiration	------------/min	
• Blood pressure	-----/--------mm Hg	
Head		
• Size and shape	Normal/shape	
• Circumference	Normocephalic/macro/microcephalic	
• Hair texture and distribution	Lustrous/coarse/sparse/normal distribution	
• Scalp	Dandruff/infestation (pediculosis)/infection	
• Fontanels: Anterior and posterior	Closed/open/enlarged/flat/depressed/bulging	
Eyes		
• Lids and lashes	Swelling/hemorrhage/lesion	
• Distance (placement)	Hypo/hypertelorism	
• Discharge movements conjunctiva	Present/absent Normal/restricted gauge	
• Vision (aquity/color)	Hemorrhage/inflammation Normal acquity/color blindness	
Ears		
• Low-set	Present/absent	
• Discharge	Present/absent	
• Preauricular tag/sinus	Present/absent	
• Microtia/macrotia/anotia	Present/absent	
• Hearing	Normal/abnormal	
Nose		
• Flaring	Present/absent	
• Discharge	Present/absent	
• Abnormality	Depressed nasal bridge/deviated nasal septum	

Contd...

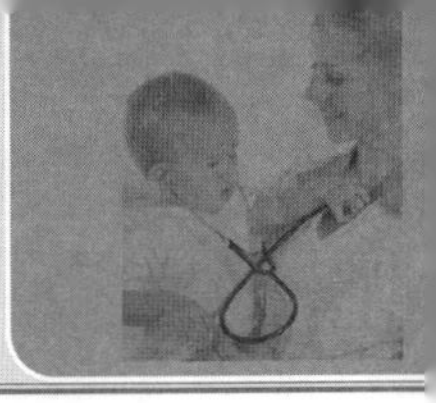

Physical features	Present in child	Any other deviation
Mouth		
• Lips—color/cleft	Pink/cyanosis/cleft	
• Palate—cleft/arch	Cleft/high arch	
• Tongue—coated, thrush	Present/absent	
• Abnormality	Macro/microglossia/drooling/mouth wide open	
• Oral mucosa	Pink/cyanosis/yellow	
• Dentition	Complete/incomplete/malocclusion/caries	
• Throat-inflammation	Present/absent	
Neck and Chest		
• **Neck**		
▪ Short/webbed	Present/absent	
▪ Lymphadenopathy	Present/absent	
▪ Birth injury/torticollis	Present/absent	
▪ Range of motion	Normal/restricted	
▪ Thyroid gland	Enlarged/normal	
▪ Tracheal deviation	Present/absent if present (R/L)	
• **Chest**		
▪ Shape and sternum	Normal/pectus carinatum/excavatum	
▪ Symmetry and movement	Equal bilateral/unequal	
▪ Work of breathing	Normal/eupnea/increased (use of accessory muscles)	
▪ Any abnormalities	Any mass/precordial bulge/heave	
▪ Circumference		
▪ Air entry	Equal bilateral/decreased (R/L)	
▪ Breath sounds	Normal/abnormal (wheeze/crackles)	
▪ Percussion	Dullness/resonance	
▪ Heart sounds	Normal S_1, S_2/murmurs/gallops/third sound	
▪ Axillary lymph nodes	Enlarged/normal	
Abdomen		
• Shape	Normal/asymmetry	
• Bowel sounds	Audible/inaudible	
• Fluid	Present/absent	
• Distension/tenderness	Present/absent	
• Girth	Hepatomegaly/splenomegaly	
• Organomegaly (liver/spleen)	Any other mass	
• Abnormality	Present/absent	

Contd...

Physical features	Present in child	Any other deviation
Perineum and Genitalia		
Male genitalia		
• Urinary meatus/stream	Central/dorsal/ventral/normal stream	
• Scrotum	Normal, pigmented/swelling	
• Testes	Descended/undescended	
• Any abnormality	Hydrocele/hernia	
Female genitalia		
• Labia minora and majora	Normal/abnormal	
• Urination	Normal/abnormal (burning)	
• Any infection	Present/absent	
Rectum and anus		
• Anal position		
• Patency/imperforation	Normal/ectopic/anterior	
• Elimination/stool pattern	Normal/abnormal	
• Any deviation	Normal/abnormal	
Extremities		
Hands and feet		
• Number of digits	Normal/poly/syn/oligodactyly	
• Nails	Pitted/spoon-shaped/splinter-hemorrhage	
• Clubbing	Present/absent	
• Creases	Simian crease/normal	
Back		
• Curvature	Normal/kyphosis/scoliosis/lordosis	
• Any tuft of hair	Present/absent	
• Pigmentation	Red rash/Mongolian spots	
• Any deviation		
Reflexes		
• Corneal		
• Pupillary		
• Abdominal		
• Biceps		
• Triceps		
• Brachioradialis		
• Knee jerk		
• Ankle jerk		
• Cremasteric (male)		
• Any other		
Impression (problems assessed)		

Nursing Diagnosis (Based on Problems Assessed)

1. __________
2. __________
3. __________
4. __________
5. __________
6. __________
7. __________
8. __________
9. __________
10. __________

Treatment Given

Physician Recommendations (Related to Care and Interventions)

____

____

____

____

____

Medicines and Fluids

Name (salt name)	Dose and route	Side effects	Nursing responsibility

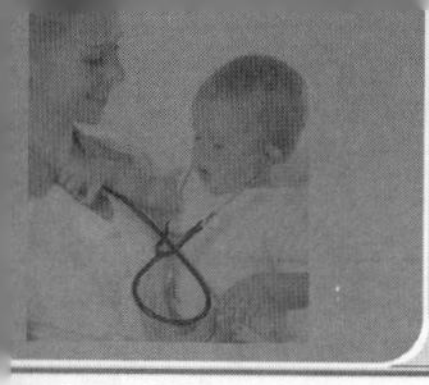

Diagnostic Tests

Test name	Findings	Remarks

Short-Term Goals

1. ______
2. ______
3. ______
4. ______
5. ______
6. ______
7. ______
8. ______
9. ______
10. ______

Long-Term Goals

1. ______
2. ______
3. ______
4. ______
5. ______
6. ______
7. ______
8. ______
9. ______
10. ______

Date/time	Nursing diagnosis	Goal	Intervention planned	Care given	Evaluation
Day 1 **Subjective data**					
Objective data					

Date/time	Nursing diagnosis	Goal	Intervention planned	Care given	Evaluation
Day 2 Subjective data					
Objective data					

Date/time	Nursing diagnosis	Goal	Intervention planned	Care given	Evaluation
Day 3 Subjective data					
Objective data					

Date/time	Nursing diagnosis	Goal	Intervention planned	Care given	Evaluation
Day 4 **Subjective data**					
Objective data					

Teacher's Signature

EVALUATION CRITERIA FOR CASE STUDY - 1

Name of Patient ______________________________

Ward/Area ______________________________

Diagnosis ______________________________

Registration No. ______________________________

Criteria	Max. marks	Marks obtained
Identification data	2	
History collection	3	
Problem assessment	5	
Nursing diagnosis framed	5	
Care planned according to priority	3	
Care implemented	2	
Description of the condition in relation to patient	3	
Description of pathophysiology and patient picture	2	
Evaluation	3	
Bibliography	2	
Total score	**30**	

Teacher's Signature

CASE STUDY - 1

Introduction of the Case

Scope and Limitation

Objectives of the Study–The Purpose of the Case Study is to:

1.
2.
3.
4.
5.

PATIENT'S PROFILE

1. Name of the Child ____________________

2. Sex ____________________

3. Mother's Name ____________________

4. Mother's Occupation and Education ____________________

5. Father's name ____________________

6. Father's Occupation and Education____________________

7. Ward/Area/Bed No. ____________________

8. Date of Birth/Age ____________________

9. Diagnosis (Medical/Surgical) ____________________

   Date of Surgery (if any) ____________________

10. Informant and Relation to Patient ____________________

11. Date of Assessment ____________________

HISTORY

Chief Complaints on Admission

Present Health History (Medical/Surgical)

Past Health History (Medical/Surgical)

Birth History (Antenatal/Intranatal/Postnatal)

Family History of Illness

Pedigree Chart

Socioeconomic Background

Food Habits–Vegetarian/Nonvegetarian/Ovo-vegetarian

Likes and Dislikes in Food Items

Allergy

Elimination Pattern

Development According to Age (Assess Milestones)

Play Activities

Growth Assessment

1. Height
2. Weight
3. Head circumference
4. Chest circumference
5. Mid upper arm circumference

Inference

Malnutrition = Actual weight/Expected weight × 100 = Grade (if any) I/II/III/IV.

Immunization History

Age	Vaccine	Given in child/date
At birth	BCG OPV Hep. B	
6 weeks	OPV Rotavac 1 Pentavac 1 (DPT + Hep. B + HiB)	
10 weeks	OPV Rotavac 1 Pentavac 1 (DPT + Hep. B + HiB)	
14 weeks	OPV Rotavac 1 Pentavac 1 (DPT + Hep. B + HiB) IPV	
9 months	Measles/MR 1, PCV booster	
16–24 months	Measles/MR 2 OPV DPT booster	
5–6 years	DPT booster	
10 and 16 years	Td	

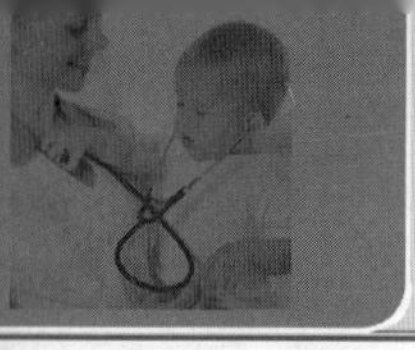

PHYSICAL ASSESSMENT

Physical features	Present in child	Any other deviation
General appearance		
• Level of consciousness	Conscious/unconscious/lethargic/stuporous	
• Posture	Normal/kyphosis/scoliosis/lordotic/guarding	
• Body built	Normal/under/over nourished/thin built	
• Facial expression	Apathy/apprehensive/depressed/normal	
• Gait	Steady/unsteady/limp	
• Ambulation	Bedridden/ambulating	
• Skin color	Pallor/cyanosis/flushed	
Vitals		
• Heart rate/pulse	--------bpm	
• Temperature	------------°C	
• Respiration	------------/min	
• Blood pressure	-----/--------mm Hg	
Head		
• Size and shape	Normal/shape	
• Circumference	Normocephalic/macro/microcephaly	
• Hair texture and distribution	Lustrous/coarse/sparse/normal distribution	
• Scalp	Dandruff/infestation (pediculosis)/infection	
• Fontanels: Anterior and Posterior	Closed/open/enlarged/flat/depressed/bulging	
Eyes		
• Lids and lashes	Swelling/hemorrhage/lesion	
• Distance (placement)	Hypo/hypertelorism	
• Discharge movements	Present/absent normal/restricted gauge	
• Conjunctiva	Hemorrhage/inflammation	
• Vision (aquity/color)	Normal acquity/color blindness	
Ears		
• Low-set	Present/absent	
• Discharge	Present/absent	
• Preauricular tag/sinus	Present/absent	
• Microtia/macrotia/anotia	Present/absent	
• Hearing	Normal/abnormal	
Nose		
• Flaring	Present/absent	
• Discharge	Present/absent	
• Abnormality	Depressed nasal bridge/deviated nasal septum	

Contd...

Physical features	Present in child	Any other deviation
Mouth		
• Lips—color/cleft	Pink/cyanosis/cleft	
• Palate—cleft/arch	Cleft/high arch	
• Tongue—coated, thrush	Present/absent	
• Abnormality	Macro/microglossia/drooling/mouth wide open	
• Oral mucosa	Pink/cyanosis/yellow	
• Dentition	Complete/incomplete/malocclusion/caries	
• Throat-inflammation	Present/absent	
Neck and Chest		
• **Neck**		
▪ Short/webbed	Present/absent	
▪ Lymphadenopathy	Present/absent	
▪ Birth injury/torticollis	Present/absent	
▪ Range of motion	Normal/restricted	
▪ Thyroid gland	Enlarged/normal	
▪ Tracheal deviation	Present/absent if present (R/L)	
• **Chest**		
▪ Shape and sternum	Normal/pectus carinatum/excavatum	
▪ Symmetry and movement	Equal bilateral/unequal	
▪ Work of breathing	Normal/eupnea/increased (use of accessory muscles)	
▪ Any abnormalities	Any mass/precordial bulge/heave	
▪ Circumference		
▪ Air entry	Equal bilateral/decreased (R/L)	
▪ Breath sounds	Normal/abnormal (wheeze/crackles)	
▪ Percussion	Dullness/resonance	
▪ Heart sounds	Normal S_1, S_2/murmurs/gallops/third sound	
▪ Axillary lymph nodes	Enlarged/normal	
Abdomen		
• Shape	Normal/asymmetry	
• Bowel sounds	Audible/inaudible	
• Fluid	Present/absent	
• Distension/tenderness	Present/absent	
• Girth	Hepatomegaly/splenomegaly	
• Organomegaly (liver/spleen)	Any other mass	
• Abnormality	Present/absent	

Contd...

Physical features	Present in child	Any other deviation
Perineum and Genitalia		
Male genitalia		
• Urinary meatus/stream	Central/dorsal/ventral/normal stream	
• Scrotum	Normal, pigmented/swelling	
• Testes	Descended/undescended	
• Any abnormality	Hydrocele/hernia	
Female genitalia		
• Labia minora and majora	Normal/abnormal	
• Urination	Normal/abnormal (burning)	
• Any infection	Present/absent	
Rectum and anus		
• Anal position		
• Patency/imperforation	Normal/ectopic/anterior	
• Elimination/stool pattern	Normal/abnormal	
• Any deviation	Normal/abnormal	
Extremities		
Hands and feet		
• Number of digits	Normal/poly/syn/oligo /dactyly	
• Nails	Pitted/spoon shaped/splinter hemorrhage	
• Clubbing	Present/absent	
• Creases	Simian crease/normal	
Back		
• Curvature	Normal/kyphosis/scoliosis/lordosis	
• Any tuft of hair	Present/absent	
• Pigmentation	Red rash/Mongolian spots	
• Any deviation		
Reflexes		
• Corneal		
• Pupillary		
• Abdominal		
• Biceps		
• Triceps		
• Brachioradialis		
• Knee jerk		
• Ankle jerk		
• Cremasteric (male)		
• Any other		
Impression (problems assessed)		

EXPLANATION OF DISEASE CONDITION

Definition

Etiology

Sl. no.	Etiology and its factors (by literature)	Inpatient

Pathophysiology

Sl. no.	Clinical manifestations (by literature)	Inpatient

Sl. no.	Diagnostic tests (by literature)	Inpatient (findings)

TREATMENT

Medical

Surgical

Nutritional Management

Supportive Management

Nursing Diagnosis (Based on Problems Assessed)

1. ______________________________

____

2. ______________________________

____

3. ______________________________

____

4. ______________________________

____

5. ______________________________

____

6. ______________________________

____

7. ______________________________

____

8. ______________________________

____

9. ______________________________

____

10. ______________________________

____

Short-Term Goals

1. ______________________________
2. ______________________________
3. ______________________________
4. ______________________________
5. ______________________________
6. ______________________________
7. ______________________________
8. ______________________________
9. ______________________________
10. ______________________________

Long-Term Goals

1. ______________________________
2. ______________________________
3. ______________________________
4. ______________________________
5. ______________________________
6. ______________________________
7. ______________________________
8. ______________________________
9. ______________________________
10. ______________________________

Medicines and Fluids

Sl. no.	Name (salt name)	Dose and route/rate	Side effects	Nursing responsibility
1.				
2.				
3.				
4.				
5.				
6.				
7.				
8.				
9.				
10.				
11.				
12.				
13.				
14.				
15.				
16.				

Date/time	Nursing diagnosis	Goal	Intervention planned	Care given	Evaluation
Day 1 **Subjective data**					
Objective data					

Date/time	Nursing diagnosis	Goal	Intervention planned	Care given	Evaluation
Day 2 Subjective data					
Objective data					

Date/time	Nursing diagnosis	Goal	Intervention planned	Care given	Evaluation
Day 3 **Subjective data**					
Objective data					

Date/time	Nursing diagnosis	Goal	Intervention planned	Care given	Evaluation
Day 4 Subjective data					
Objective data					

Date/time	Nursing diagnosis	Goal	Intervention planned	Care given	Evaluation
Day 5 **Subjective data**					
Objective data					

Date/time	Nursing diagnosis	Goal	Intervention planned	Care given	Evaluation
Day 6 **Subjective data**					
Objective data					

Teacher's Signature

Discharge Summary

Bibliography

1.
2.
3.
4.
5.
6.
7.
8.
9.
10.

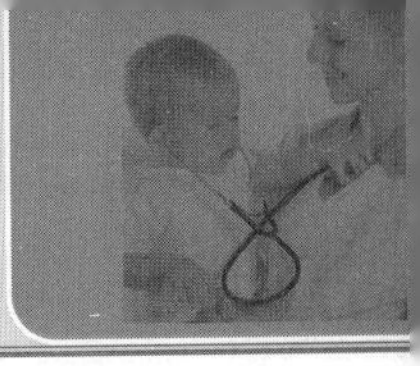

EVALUATION CRITERIA FOR CASE STUDY – 2

Name of Patient ______________________________________

Ward/Area ______________________________________

Diagnosis ______________________________________

Registration No. ______________________________________

Criteria	Max. marks	Marks obtained
Identification data	2	
History collection	3	
Problem assessment	5	
Nursing diagnosis framed	5	
Care planned according to priority	3	
Care implemented	2	
Description of the condition in relation to patient	3	
Description of pathophysiology and patient picture	2	
Evaluation	3	
Bibliography	2	
Total score	**30**	

Teacher's Signature

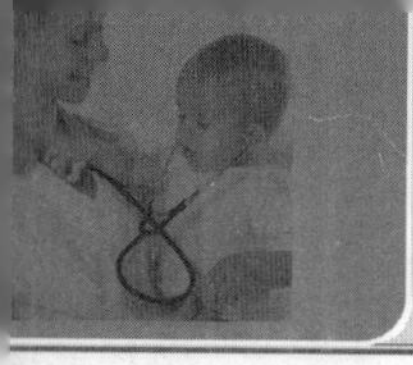

CASE STUDY - 2

Introduction of the Case

Scope and Limitation

Objectives of the Study–The Purpose of the Case Study is to:

1.
2.
3.
4.
5.

PATIENT'S PROFILE

1. Name of the Child ______________________________

2. Sex ______________________________

3. Mother's Name ______________________________

4. Mother's Occupation and Education ______________________________

5. Father's Name ______________________________

6. Father's Occupation and Education ______________________________

7. Ward/Area/Bed no. ______________________________

8. Date of Birth/Age ______________________________

9. Diagnosis (Medical/Surgical) ______________________________

   Date of Surgery (if any) ______________________________

10. Informant and Relation to Patient ______________________________

11. Date of Assessment ______________________________

HISTORY

Chief Complaints on Admission

Present Health History (Medical/Surgical)

Past Health History (Medical/Surgical)

Birth History (Antenatal/Intranatal/Postnatal)

Family History of Illness

Pedigree Chart

Socioeconomic Background

Food Habits–Vegetarian/Nonvegetarian/Ovo-vegetarian

Likes and Dislikes in Food Items

Allergy

Elimination Pattern

Development According to Age (Assess Milestones)

Play Activities

Growth Assessment

1. **Height** ____________________
2. **Weight** ____________________
3. **Head circumference** ____________________
4. **Chest circumference** ____________________
5. **Mid upper arm circumference** ____________________
6. **Inference** ____________________

Malnutrition = Actual weight/Expected weight × 100 = Grade (if any) I/II/III/IV.

Immunization History

Age	Vaccine	Given in child/date
At birth	BCG OPV Hep. B	
6 weeks	OPV Rotavac 1 Pentavac 1 (DPT + Hep. B + HiB)	
10 weeks	OPV Rotavac 1 Pentavac 1 (DPT + Hep. B + HiB)	
14 weeks	OPV Rotavac 1 Pentavac 1 (DPT + Hep. B + HiB) IPV	
9 months	Measles/MR 1, PCV booster	
16–24 months	Measles/MR 2 OPV DPT booster	
5–6 years	DPT booster	
10 and 16 years	Td	

PHYSICAL ASSESSMENT

Physical features	Present in child	Any other deviation
General appearance		
• Level of consciousness	Conscious/unconscious/lethargic/stuporous	
• Posture	Normal/kyphosis/scoliosis/lordotic/guarding	
• Body built	Normal/under/overnourished/thin built	
• Facial expression	Apathy/apprehensive/depressed/normal	
• Gait	Steady/unsteady/limp	
• Ambulation	Bedridden/ambulating	
• Skin color	Pallor/cyanosis/flushed	
Vitals		
• Heart rate/pulse	--------bpm	
• Temperature	------------°C	
• Respiration	------------/min	
• Blood pressure	-----/--------mm Hg	
Head		
• Size and shape	Normal/shape	
• Circumference	Normocephalic/macro/microcephalic	
• Hair texture and distribution	Lustrous/coarse/sparse/normal distribution	
• Scalp	Dandruff/infestation (pediculosis)/infection	
• Fontanels: Anterior and Posterior	Closed/open/enlarged/flat/depressed/bulging	
Eyes		
• Lids and lashes	Swelling/hemorrhage/lesion	
• Distance (placement)	Hypo/hypertelorism present/absent	
• Discharge movements	Normal/restricted gauge	
• Conjunctiva	Hemorrhage/inflammation	
• Vision (aquity/color)	Normal acquity/color blindness	
Ears		
• Low-set	Present/absent	
• Discharge	Present/absent	
• Preauricular tag/sinus	Present/absent	
• Microtia/macrotia/anotia	Present/absent	
• Hearing	Normal/abnormal	
Nose		
• Flaring	Present/absent	
• Discharge	Present/absent	
• Abnormality	Depressed nasal bridge/deviated nasal septum	

Contd...

Physical features	Present in child	Any other deviation
Mouth		
• Lips—color/cleft	Pink/cyanosis/cleft	
• Palate—cleft/arch	Cleft/high arch	
• Tongue—coated, thrush	Present/absent	
• Abnormality	Macro/microglossia/drooling/mouth wide open	
• Oral mucosa	Pink/cyanosis/yellow	
• Dentition	Complete/incomplete/malocclusion/caries	
• Throat-inflammation	Present/absent	
Neck and Chest		
• **Neck**		
▪ Short/webbed	Present/absent	
▪ Lymphadenopathy	Present/absent	
▪ Birth injury/torticollis	Present/absent	
▪ Range of motion	Normal/restricted	
▪ Thyroid gland	Enlarged/normal	
▪ Tracheal deviation	Present/absent if present (R/L)	
• **Chest**		
▪ Shape and sternum	Normal/pectus carinatum/excavatum	
▪ Symmetry and movement	Equal bilateral/unequal	
▪ Work of breathing	Normal/eupnea/increased (use of accessory muscles)	
▪ Any abnormalities	Any mass/precordial bulge/heave	
▪ Circumference		
▪ Air entry	Equal bilateral/decreased (R/L)	
▪ Breath sounds	Normal/abnormal (wheeze/crackles)	
▪ Percussion	Dullness/resonance	
▪ Heart sounds	Normal S_1, S_2/murmurs/gallops/third sound	
▪ Axillary lymph nodes	Enlarged/normal	
Abdomen		
• Shape	Normal/asymmetry	
• Bowel sounds	Audible/inaudible	
• Fluid	Present/absent	
• Distension /tenderness	Present/absent	
• Girth	Hepatomegaly/splenomegaly	
• Organomegaly (liver/spleen)	Any other mass	
• Abnormality	Present/absent	

Contd...

Physical features	Present in child	Any other deviation
Perineum and Genitalia		
Male genitalia		
• Urinary meatus/stream	Central/dorsal/ventral/normal stream	
• Scrotum	Normal, pigmented/swelling	
• Testes	Descended/undescended	
• Any abnormality	Hydrocele/hernia	
Female genitalia		
• Labia minora and majora	Normal/abnormal	
• Urination	Normal/abnormal (burning)	
• Any infection	Present/absent	
Rectum and anus		
• Anal position		
• Patency/imperforation	Normal/ectopic/anterior	
• Elimination/stool pattern	Normal/abnormal	
• Any deviation	Normal/abnormal	
Extremities		
Hands and feet		
• Number of digits	Normal/poly/syn/oligo /dactyly	
• Nails	Pitted/spoon shaped/splinter hemorrhage	
• Clubbing	Present/absent	
• Creases	Simian crease/normal	
Back		
• Curvature	Normal/kyphosis/scoliosis/lordosis	
• Any tuft of hair	Present/absent	
• Pigmentation	Red rash/Mongolian spots	
• Any deviation		
Reflexes		
• Corneal		
• Pupillary		
• Abdominal		
• Biceps		
• Triceps		
• Brachioradialis		
• Knee jerk		
• Ankle jerk		
• Cremasteric (male)		
• Any other		
Impression (problems assessed)		

EXPLANATION OF DISEASE CONDITION

Definition

Etiology

Sl. no.	Etiology and its factors (by literature)	Inpatient

Pathophysiology

Sl. no.	Clinical manifestations (by literature)	Inpatient

Sl. no.	Diagnostic tests (by literature)	Inpatient (findings)

TREATMENT

Medical

Surgical

Nutritional Management

Supportive Management

Nursing Diagnosis (Based on Problems Assessed)

1. __________

2. __________

3. __________

4. __________

5. __________

6. __________

7. __________

8. __________

9. __________

10. __________

Short-Term Goals

1. ____________________
2. ____________________
3. ____________________
4. ____________________
5. ____________________
6. ____________________
7. ____________________
8. ____________________
9. ____________________
10. ____________________

Long-Term Goals

1. ____________________
2. ____________________
3. ____________________
4. ____________________
5. ____________________
6. ____________________
7. ____________________
8. ____________________
9. ____________________
10. ____________________

Medicines and Fluids

Sl. no.	Name (salt name)	Dose and route/rate	Side effects	Nursing responsibility
1.				
2.				
3.				
4.				
5.				
6.				
7.				
8.				
9.				
10.				
11.				
12.				
13.				
14.				
15.				
16.				

Date/time	Nursing diagnosis	Goal	Intervention planned	Care given	Evaluation
Day 1 Subjective data					
Objective data					

Date/time	Nursing diagnosis	Goal	Intervention planned	Care given	Evaluation
Day 2 Subjective data					
Objective data					

Date/time	Nursing diagnosis	Goal	Intervention planned	Care given	Evaluation
Day 3 Subjective data					
Objective data					

Date/time	Nursing diagnosis	Goal	Intervention planned	Care given	Evaluation
Day 4 Subjective data					
Objective data					

Date/time	Nursing diagnosis	Goal	Intervention planned	Care given	Evaluation
Day 5 **Subjective data**					
Objective data					

Date/time	Nursing diagnosis	Goal	Intervention planned	Care given	Evaluation
Day 6 Subjective data					
Objective data					

Teacher's Signature

Discharge Summary

Bibliography

1.
2.
3.
4.
5.
6.
7.
8.
9.
10.

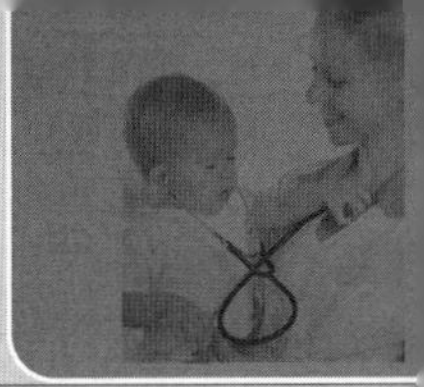

EVALUATION CRITERIA FOR HEALTH TALK – 1

Topic ________________________________

Audience and number ________________________________

Date/time ________________________________

Location ________________________________

AV aids used ________________________________

Criteria	Max. marks	Marks obtained
Introduction of topic	5	
Content adequacy	5	
Presentation (voice, language), use of AV aids	5	
Group feedback	5	
Answered queries	5	
Total	**25**	

Teacher's Signature

CONTENT FOR HEALTH TALK

Topic: ______________________________

Content: ______________________________

EVALUATION CRITERIA FOR HEALTH TALK – 2

Topic ______________________________

Audience and number ______________________________

Date/time ______________________________

Location ______________________________

AV aids used ______________________________

Criteria	Max. marks	Marks obtained
Introduction of topic	5	
Content adequacy	5	
Presentation (voice, language), use of AV aids	5	
Group feedback	5	
Answered queries	5	
Total	**25**	

Teacher's Signature

CONTENT FOR HEALTH TALK

Topic: ______________________________

Content: ______________________________

NANDA–APPROVED NURSING DIAGNOSES 2021–23

Domain 1: Health Promotion

Class 1. Health Awareness

- Decreased diversional activity engagement
- Readiness for enhanced health literacy
- Sedentary lifestyle

Class 2. Health Management

- Risk for elopement attempt
- Frail elderly syndrome
- Risk for frail elderly syndrome
- Readiness for enhanced exercise engagement
- Deficient community health
- Risk-prone health behavior
- Ineffective health maintenance behaviors
- Ineffective health self-management
- Readiness for enhanced health self-management
- Ineffective family health self-management
- Ineffective home maintenance behaviors
- Risk for ineffective home maintenance behaviors
- Readiness for enhanced home maintenance behaviors
- Ineffective protection

Domain 2: Nutrition

Class 1. Ingestion

- Imbalanced nutrition: less than body requirements
- Readiness for enhanced nutrition
- Insufficient breast milk production
- Ineffective breastfeeding
- Interrupted breastfeeding
- Readiness for enhanced breastfeeding
- Ineffective adolescent eating dynamics
- Ineffective child eating dynamics
- Ineffective infant feeding dynamics
- Obesity
- Overweight
- Risk for overweight
- Ineffective infant suck-swallow response
- Impaired swallowing

Class 2. Digestion

None at present time

Class 3. Absorption

None at present time

Class 4. Metabolism

- Risk for unstable blood glucose level
- Neonatal hyperbilirubinemia
- Risk for neonatal hyperbilirubinemia
- Risk for impaired liver function
- Risk for metabolic syndrome

Class 5. Hydration

- Risk for electrolyte imbalance
- Risk for imbalanced fluid volume
- Deficient fluid volume
- Risk for deficient fluid volume
- Excess fluid volume

Domain 3: Elimination and Exchange

Class 1. Urinary Function

- Disability-associated urinary incontinence
- Impaired urinary elimination
- Mixed urinary incontinence
- Stress urinary incontinence
- Urge urinary incontinence
- Risk for urge urinary incontinence
- Urinary retention
- Risk for urinary retention

Class 2. Gastrointestinal Function

- Constipation
- Risk for constipation
- Perceived constipation
- Chronic functional constipation
- Risk for chronic functional constipation
- Impaired bowel continence
- Diarrhea
- Dysfunctional gastrointestinal motility
- Risk for dysfunctional gastrointestinal motility

Class 3. Integumentary Function

None at this time

Class 4. Respiratory Function

Impaired gas exchange

Domain 4: Activity/Rest

Class 1. Sleep/Rest Insomnia

- Sleep deprivation
- Readiness for enhanced sleep
- Disturbed sleep pattern

Class 2. Activity/Exercise

- Decreased activity tolerance
- Risk for decreased activity tolerance
- Risk for disuse syndrome
- Impaired bed mobility
- Impaired physical mobility
- Impaired wheelchair mobility
- Impaired sitting
- Impaired standing
- Impaired transfer ability
- Impaired walking

Class 3. Energy Balance

- Imbalanced energy field
- Fatigue
- Wandering

Class 4. Cardiovascular/Pulmonary Responses

- Ineffective breathing pattern
- Decreased cardiac output
- Risk for decreased cardiac output
- Risk for impaired cardiovascular function
- Ineffective lymphedema self-management
- Risk for ineffective lymphedema self-management
- Impaired spontaneous ventilation
- Risk for unstable blood pressure
- Risk for thrombosis
- Risk for decreased cardiac tissue perfusion
- Risk for ineffective cerebral tissue perfusion
- Ineffective peripheral tissue perfusion
- Risk for ineffective peripheral tissue perfusion
- Dysfunctional ventilatory weaning response
- Dysfunctional adult ventilatory weaning response

Class 5. Self-Care

- Bathing self-care deficit
- Dressing self-care deficit
- Feeding self-care deficit
- Toileting self-care deficit
- Readiness for enhanced self-care
- Self-neglect

Domain 5: Perception/Cognition

Class 1. Attention

Unilateral neglect

Class 2. Orientation

This class does not currently contain any diagnoses

Class 3. Sensation/Perception

This class does not currently contain any diagnoses

Class 4. Cognition

- Acute confusion
- Risk for acute confusion
- Chronic confusion
- Labile emotional control
- Ineffective impulse control
- Deficient knowledge
- Readiness for enhanced knowledge
- Impaired memory
- Disturbed thought process

Class 5. Communication

- Readiness for enhanced communication
- Impaired verbal communication

Domain 6: Self-Perception

Class 1. Self-Concept

- Hopelessness
- Readiness for enhanced hope
- Risk for compromised human dignity
- Disturbed personal identity
- Risk for disturbed personal identity
- Readiness for enhanced self-concept

Class 2. Self-Esteem

- Chronic low self-esteem
- Risk for chronic low self-esteem
- Situational low self-esteem
- Risk for situational low self-esteem

Class 3. Body Image

Disturbed body image

Domain 7: Role Relationship

Class 1. Caregiving Roles

- Impaired parenting
- Risk for impaired parenting
- Readiness for enhanced parenting
- Caregiver role strain
- Risk for caregiver role strain

Class 2. Family Relationships

- Risk for impaired attachment
- Disturbed family identity syndrome
- Risk for disturbed family identity syndrome
- Dysfunctional family processes
- Interrupted family processes
- Readiness for enhanced family processes

Class 3. Role Performance

- Ineffective relationship
- Risk for ineffective relationship
- Readiness for enhanced relationship
- Parental role conflict
- Ineffective role performance
- Impaired social interaction

Domain 8: Sexuality

Class 1. Sexual Identity

This class does not currently contain any diagnosis

Class 2. Sexual Function

- Sexual dysfunction
- Ineffective sexuality pattern

Class 3. Rcproduction

- Ineffective childbearing process
- Risk for ineffective childbearing process
- Readiness for enhanced childbearing process
- Risk for disturbed maternal-fetal dyad

Domain 9: Coping/Stress Tolerance

Class 1. Post-Trauma Responses

- Risk for complicated immigration transition
- Post-trauma syndrome
- Risk for post-trauma syndrome
- Rape-trauma syndrome
- Relocation stress syndrome
- Risk for relocation stress syndrome

Class 2. Coping Responses

- Ineffective activity planning
- Risk for ineffective activity planning
- Anxiety
- Defensive coping
- Ineffective coping
- Readiness for enhanced coping
- Ineffective community coping
- Readiness for enhanced community coping
- Compromised family coping
- Disabled family coping
- Readiness for enhanced family coping
- Death anxiety
- Ineffective denial
- Fear
- Maladaptive grieving
- Risk for maladaptive grieving
- Readiness for enhanced grieving
- Impaired mood regulation
- Powerlessness
- Risk for powerlessness
- Readiness for enhanced power
- Impaired resilience
    - Risk for impaired resilience
    - Readiness for enhanced resilience
    - Chronic sorrow
    - Stress overload

Class 3. Neurobehavioral Stress

- Acute substance withdrawal syndrome
- Risk for acute substance withdrawal syndrome
- Autonomic dysreflexia
- Risk for autonomic dysreflexia
- Neonatal abstinence syndrome
- Disorganized infant behavior
- Risk for disorganized infant behavior
- Readiness for enhanced organized infant behavior

Domain 10: Life Principles

Class 1. Values

This class does not currently contain any diagnosis

Class 2. Beliefs

Readiness for enhanced spiritual well-being

Class 3. Value/Belief/Action Congruence

- Readiness for enhanced decision-making
- Decisional conflict
- Impaired emancipated decision-making
- Risk for impaired emancipated decision-making
- Readiness for enhanced emancipated decision-making
- Moral distress
- Impaired religiosity
- Risk for impaired religiosity
- Readiness for enhanced religiosity
- Spiritual distress
- Risk for spiritual distress

Domain 11: Safety/Protection

Class 1. Infection

- Risk for infection
- Risk for surgical site infection

Class 2. Physical Injury

- Ineffective airway clearance
- Risk for aspiration
- Risk for bleeding
- Impaired dentition
- Risk for dry eye
- Ineffective dry eye self-management
- Risk for dry mouth
- Risk for adult falls
- Risk for child falls
- Risk for injury
- Risk for corneal injury
- Nipple-areolar complex injury
- Risk for nipple-areolar complex injury
- Risk for urinary tract injury
- Risk for perioperative positioning injury
- Risk for thermal injury
- Impaired oral mucous membrane integrity
- Risk for impaired oral mucous membrane integrity
- Risk for peripheral neurovascular dysfunction
- Risk for physical trauma
- Risk for vascular trauma
- Adult pressure injury
- Risk for adult pressure injury
- Child pressure injury
- Risk for child pressure injury
- Neonatal pressure injury
- Risk for neonatal pressure injury
- Risk for shock
- Impaired skin integrity
- Risk for impaired skin integrity
- Risk for sudden infant death
- Risk for suffocation
- Delayed surgical recovery
- Risk for delayed surgical recovery
- Impaired tissue integrity
- Risk for impaired tissue integrity

Class 3. Violence

- Risk for female genital mutilation
- Risk for other-directed violence
- Risk for self-directed violence
- Self-mutilation
- Risk for self-mutilation
- Risk for suicidal behavior

Class 4. Environmental Hazards

- Contamination
- Risk for contamination
- Risk for occupational injury
- Risk for poisoning

Class 5. Defensive Processes

- Risk for adverse reaction to iodinated contrast media
- Risk for allergy reaction
- Risk for latex allergy reaction

Class 6. Thermoregulation

- Hyperthermia
- Hypothermia
- Risk for hypothermia
- Neonatal hypothermia
- Risk for neonatal hypothermia
- Risk for perioperative hypothermia
- Ineffective thermoregulation
- Risk for ineffective thermoregulation

Domain 12: Comfort

Class 1. Physical Comfort

- Impaired comfort
- Readiness for enhanced comfort

- Nausea
- Acute pain
- Chronic pain
- Chronic pain syndrome
- Labor pain

Class 2. Environmental Comfort

- Impaired comfort
- Readiness for enhanced comfort

Class 3. Social Comfort

- Impaired comfort
- Readiness for enhanced comfort
- Risk for loneliness
- Social isolation

Domain 13: Growth/Development

Class 1. Growth

This class does not currently contain any diagnosis

Class 2. Development

- Delayed child development
- Risk for delayed child development
- Delayed infant motor development
- Risk for delayed infant motor